Ethical Problems in the Nurse-Patient Relationship

Catherine P. Murphy
Boston College

Howard Hunter
Tufts University

Allyn and Bacon, Inc.
Boston   London   Sydney   Toronto

Library of Congress Cataloging in Publication Data
Main entry under title:

Ethical problems in the nurse-patient relationship.

Includes index.
1. Nursing ethics. 2. Nurse and patient. I. Murphy,
Catherine. II. Hunter, Howard.
RT85.E832 *1983*   174'.2   81–22847
ISBN 0-205-07762-5   AACR2

Managing Editor: Hiram G. Howard

Printed in the United States of America.

10 9 8 7 6 5 4 3 2 1   87 86 85 84 83 82

For

Mary Lyne Murphy

James Murphy

Jesse Charles Hunter

Zelva Hunter Steiner

Contents

Section IV   Issues in the Nurse–Patient Relationship   149

Appendices

Contributors

Mila A. Aroskar
Department of Public Health Nursing
School of Public Health
University of Minnesota

Bertram Bandman
Department of Philosophy
Long Island University

Elsie Bandman
Hunter College–Bellevue School of
    Nursing
City University of New York

Anne J. Davis
School of Nursing
University of California,
    San Francisco

Sally Gadow
College of Medicine
University of Florida, Gainesville

Joseph M. Healey
School of Medicine
University of Connecticut
    Health Center

Howard Hunter
Department of Religion
Tufts University

Alasdair MacIntyre
Department of Philosophy
Vanderbilt University

Elizabeth M. Maloney
Department of Nursing Education
Teachers College
Columbia University

Diane Deegan McCrann
College of Nursing
Villanova University

Catherine Murphy
School of Nursing
Boston College

Robert Neville
The Stony Brook Center for
    Religious Studies
State University of New York at
    Stony Brook

Linda O'Brien
College of Nursing
University of Delaware

Partricia A. O'Neil
Department of Health and Hospitals
City of Boston

Gary S. Orgel
Department of Philosophy
Boston University

Jay Schulkin
Institute of Neurological Sciences
University of Pennsylvania

Sandra Reed Sweezy
Beth Israel Hospital, Boston

Preface

In relating to patients, today's nurse is confronted with unprecedented moral problems while, at the same time, she is faced with a professional identity crisis. It is the purpose of this book to examine a number of these moral problems and to consider the nursing profession from the perspectives of practicing nurses, nurse educators, and academic specialists who share a concern for the issues that nurses are facing.

Issues that affect everyone who is concerned for health and for the quality of health care in our society are addressed in this book. Its subjects are of special interest to members of the nursing profession, including students of nursing, practicing nurses, and nursing educators. They should also be of interest to other members of the health care professions since the essays consider problems encountered frequently in health care practice.

We wish to acknowledge with appreciation the assistance we have received in the preparation of this volume. We are grateful to the contributors for their unfailing cooperation and generous support. Some of the essays in this volume are written by authors who participated in the Massachusetts phase of a larger project entitled "Nursing and the Humanities: A Public Dialogue." This project was supported equally by grants from four state humanities committees of the National Endowment for the Humanities: The Connecticut Humanities Council (P7710–G 7716); The Massachusetts Foundation for Humanities and Public Policy (May 7–2); The New York Council for the Humanities (77–301); and the Rhode Island Committee for the Humanities (767721). The project director of the four state consortium was Stuart F. Spicker of Connecticut and the state coordinators were: Elsie Bandman, Bertram Bandman, and Peter Williams of New York; Lois Monteiro and Sheri Smith of Rhode Island; Anne Donnelly and Lisa Newton of Connecticut; and Howard Hunter and Catherine Murphy of Massachusetts.

To Nathaniel Reed, Executive Director of the Massachusetts Foundation for Humanities and Public Policy we wish to offer a special word of thanks for his enthusiasm and encouragement for this project. Finally, we are greatly indebted to Mrs. Deborah Walsh, Secretary of the Department of Religion at Tufts University, for her patient and gracious assistance throughout every phase of this project.

Introduction

Today's nurse practices in an environment which is vastly more complicated culturally, technologically, and bureaucratically than any of her nursing sisters of the past, even the very recent past, have known. Culturally, she must treat persons of widely varying convictions about the meaning of health and sickness. She treats persons who are not so inclined as in the past to remain the silent beneficiaries of, or as some might put it victims of, whatever passes for sufficient health care within the various health care professions. Technologically, she practices within a context in which machines threaten to dominate and to determine moral and ethical decisions. Bureaucratically, she is still expected to accept a position of subordination in a society in which all such subordination is under sustained and vigorous attack, especially subordination that does not appear to further the objectives of the nurse in helping patients and which, to make matters worse, is apparently associated with the presuppositions and practices of a patriarchal culture. Today's nurse may expect to have to function professionally for some if not all of her career in a context of bureaucratic complexity in which she must somehow accommodate her own personal and professional ideals to those of another health care profession, medicine, and those of an institution, the hospital.

To practice nursing today in such an environment would be difficult for the most mature, thoroughly prepared, and self-reliant professional individual. It is clear that the nursing profession is fortunate to have considerable numbers of members with precisely these characteristics. Yet, for others the environment of today's nursing practice precipitates a crisis of identity. The nurse is forced, often quite literally, to ask herself just who she is, what it means to be a nurse, what her obligations are, and to whom she owes her loyalties. Simple answers to these questions, once perhaps adequate if not satisfying, will no longer do. It is not enough for today's nurse to content herself with the self-assurance that she means well in her desire to help others in need. She has to face the fact that her practice will take place in a complex situation not of her making. She has to see that all traditional and conventional systems and solutions to problems are under critical scrutiny. She has to acknowledge that at times her understanding of the patient's needs may well differ from the understanding that a physician has. She must determine whether she is obligated more to the patient than to the physician or to the institution in which she practices. In dealing with problems patients present she soon has to confront the problem she herself presents: who is she? what are her values? what is her own understanding of illness and of health? what is her vocation, her calling? These are the questions of identity.

To have a crisis of identity is not itself a sickness. On the contrary, not to have one is a sickness, for until one has a crisis of identity, one is simply accepting the stereotyped picture someone else has of one's self. Clearly, it is to the advantage of those whose loyalties and interests are in maintaining the status quo to keep nurses from challenging prevailing procedural and professional patterns. Be that as it may, it is the purpose of this book to challenge each nurse and nursing student to reflect as seriously as she can upon the moral and ethical issues her relationship to patients presents and, further, to give her most sustained and thoughtful reflection on her own identity as a nurse.

Section I begins with Catherine Murphy's critical examination of three current models of the nurse–patient relationship. Tracing the historical evolution of these models, she shows the impact of each model upon the ethical decision making process within nursing. Her essay offers recommendations for reform in current education for nursing and for today's nursing practice.

Howard Hunter presents an interpretation of nursing as a humane profession. Seeing the nurse as the primary caring agent in the health care professions, he interprets the place of studies in the humanities for the humane nurse.

The philosophical foundations for the nurse as advocate for the patient are developed by Sally Gadow. She reviews historic ideal concepts of nursing and rejects both paternalism and patients' rights advocacy in favor of advocacy for the whole person. She terms such an approach "existential advocacy" and develops a comprehensive rationale for it.

Section II opens with an essay by Anne Davis in which she analyses the social organization and the structure of the hospital. She closely examines the sociology of ethics in hospitals and considers the crucial question of collective bargaining and strikes within the nursing profession. She offers a number of penetratingly critical questions regarding the current practices of medical and hospital personnel.

Doctors cure, nurse care, or so a familiar statement has it. But Alasdair MacIntyre questions whether the terms "cure" and "care" have been adequately defined and differentiated. He notes the inadequacies of the present nurse-physician relationship and stresses the role of the nurse as an interpreter between physician and patient. He questions the appropriateness of the present nurse-physician relationships.

If one accepts the concept of the nurse as patient advocate, Elsie Bandman asks, who will be the nurse's advocate? She sees today's hospitals as an industry having many of the characteristics of complex and bureaucratic big business. Examining models of the nurse–patient relationship she concludes that no one model supplies all the answers to the issues and dilemmas of patient and nursing rights. In answering Murphy's and MacIntyre's questions as to whom the nurse is responsible, she holds that the nurse is responsible to the patient, the physician, and the hospital—all three, and that all three are responsible for seeing that there is justice for all.

One area in which nurses face moral problems in their professional practice is in connection with patients' rights. Bertram Bandman opens Section III with a detailed discussion of this problem. Examining theories of rights in both historical and contemporary contexts, he considers a practical application of rights in a specific well-known case in which the rights of the nurse, the patient, and the physician were seen to be in conflict.

The formation of the concept of patients' rights and its implications for nursing education and nursing practice are considered by Joseph Healey. He argues that greater awareness of these matters should strengthen the nurse in her awareness of her own profession as well as provide eventual benefits to the patients for whom she cares.

Nurses are deeply involved in another type of care in which moral problems frequently manifest themselves. This is the problem of caring for persons who are terminally ill. Gary Orgel reflects upon the nurse's situation in such cases. He is specifically concerned with the question of the patient's right to know of her or his own condition. Orgel explores the legal and philosophical dimensions of this issue and clearly demonstrates the complexity of the problems involved. He notes that all moral judgments are social judgments. He urges that nurses, individually and collectively, struggle ceaselessly to play an equal role in the decision making process with regard to informing the patient about her or his condition.

Individual autonomy and community responsibility are the focus of Mila Aroskar's discussion as to whether the patient has a right to reject treatment. Increasingly we see a concern for the rights of individuals in this area and Aroskar's concern is to note the crucial influence of the nurse in the process of the patient's decision making. She emphasizes the importance of humane concern and compassion on the part of the nurse in this process.

Elizabeth Maloney opens Section IV with a discussion of the problems nurses face today in the administration of drugs. Others prescribe, nurses administer. What of the nurse's moral concerns regarding the use and the abuse of drugs? Where are her obligations? What are some of the problems the nurse faces and what should be her response to the moral questions drug administration poses?

Elizabeth Maloney examines the ethics of drug administration from the nurse's perspective. She develops the position that the nurse's willingness to participate in the act of drug administration has to be considered on a case-to-case basis and with a careful consideration of the ethical and moral issues involved. Jay Schulkin and Robert Neville consider further the dilemmas of drug administration with specific reference to behavior control. They see the problem as requiring concern not only for the role of nurses but of physicians and patients as well.

Case studies by practicing nurses presenting specific moral and ethical problems which nurses must be prepared to face conclude the volume. Diane Deegan McCrann considers a case in which a medical staff member ordered the administration of a behavior modifying drug in order to perform a medical procedure against the expressed wishes of the patient. McCrann argues that such a procedure is immoral and that the nurse is under a moral obligation not to participate in it.

Patricia O'Neill examines the ethical issues facing nurses who are involved in the administration of placebos, harmless substances which the patient is given with the understanding that he or she is receiving something of genuine therapeutic value. She questions whether it is appropriate for nurses to participate in the administration of such materials.

The final essays are concerned with moral dilemmas which are especially poignant as well as complex. The first deals with the allocation of scarce health care resources. Nurses practicing today will find increasing numbers of situations similar to the one that Linda O'Brien describes. She shows how nurses are required to perform a most delicate and sensitive task of interpreting health care policies which make available health resources to some while denying them to others. Her essay presents a specific case in which we see the large issues of governmental health care policy, medical diagnoses, ethics of social responsibility, and individual moral decisions coming to a focus. As in so many other instances discussed throughout this book, the nurse is seen as obligated not only to understand these issues but to translate them into terms accessible to patients in great need and often in great distress.

Another moral issue with which nurses today are forced to deal is the use of human subjects for scientific and medical research. Sandra Reed Sweezy provides a study in which the ethics of research involving the informed consent of the subjects is the focus. She provides a conceptual basis for the conclusion that it is morally wrong to use human subjects even though the goal of the research may be the commendable desire to advance human knowledge.

The essays in this book stand on their own, for each considers a different aspect of the nursing profession and the moral and ethical dilemmas it faces today. But taken together the essays offer a compelling demonstration of the centrality of nursing to the health care system. They show that nurses must see themselves and be seen as primary providers of that humane and moral care that alone gives life—and health—its meaning and its justification.

I

Foundations of the Nursing Profession

This section is concerned with what we may call the foundations of the nursing profession. By foundations we mean the basic ideas nurses have of their profession. We mean also the model or ideal nurse which practicing nurses aspire to become. The definition of the word "profession" is more difficult, since there is no universally accepted understanding of what is required to characterize certain activities as professions. Upon one point there is general agreement, however, and that is that a principal characteristic of a profession is that its practitioners act as morally responsible agents freely accepting of and committed to the purposes of the professional group.

To be a professional person requires that one be personally involved not only in the performance of the obligations of the profession but also in critically evaluating the appropriateness of that performance in the light of the profession's purposes. A professional person is not allowed the dubious satisfaction of simply doing a job or of following orders without further reflection. To be a professional person is to accept the difficult and demanding need to think through the implications of every phase of one's professional activities. It is to accept the necessity of forming for one's self the model or ideal practitioner and to judge one's performance by it.

Whether or not nursing is a profession is ultimately decided by the thoughts and actions of nurses themselves. If nurses uncritically accept whatever role is thrust upon them, they are not professionals but simply employees. It is safe to say that the impetus to achieve professional status must come from within the ranks of practicing nurses. This section begins with an essay by an experienced nurse who has given considerable attention in recent years as a nursing educator to the models available to the nursing profession and to the ethical problems that nurses face. This essay is followed by one written by a professor in another of the helping professions who sees nursing as a humane profession. The section concludes with another essay by a philosopher of health care familiar with the practical aspects as well as the philosophical foundations of nursing practice and the nursing profession.

How should the nurse relate to the patient? This deceptively simple question is perhaps the most fundamental one confronting nurses throughout their careers. It is also one of the most difficult questions to answer, for there are significantly different but equally strongly defended views on the subject. The Socratic suggestion that the unexamined life is not worth living may be extended to the profession of nursing. It may be too much to say that the unexamined practice of nursing is not worth doing, but nurses who enter uncritically and unreflectively into any given nursing situation can face conditions that they may find quite unacceptable.

It is important for the nurse to be able to articulate her own understanding of the ideal model of nursing and of the ideal context in which she practices. Catherine Murphy's essay opens this book by examining alternative models of the nurse–patient relationship. She explores the implications of each model for the practical area of making ethical decisions, and she suggests that the time for serious and far-reaching reform both in the preparation nurses receive and in the contexts in which they carry out their profession is upon us.

I

Models of the Nurse-Patient Relationship

Catherine P. Murphy

The contemporary idealized role of the nurse in health care is one of a patient advocate who creates an environment that supports and enables the patient to maintain his or her own autonomy and dignity as a person. The notion of the nurse as a human rights advocate in the health care system is an admirable ideal to strive for, but the barriers that stand in the way of the nurse are indeed staggering. Before we as nurses can begin to engage in serious moral discourse and deal with specific ethical issues in health care, we must come to grips with the very complex social and psychological forces that prevent the nurse from acting on moral convictions as an advocate for the patient.[1]

The ethical perspective in nursing practice has changed over the years in relation to social thinking and the values of the times. The impact of spiritual forces in the middle ages fostered respect for the dignity of personhood and the humanistic care of the sick and needy.[2] The Nightingale era set into motion a reformation in nursing that was concerned with humane care and social reform. The current century in many ways can be seen as a dark period in the history of nursing ethics. The deterioration in the nurse–patient relationship can be attributed to what I perceive to be two main social forces—the effect of technology and the bureaucratic industrialization of health care institutions.

Adapted from "Ethical Aspects of Decision Making in Nursing" by Catherine P. Murphy published in *Political, Social and Educational Forces in Nursing: Impact of Social Forces.* New York: National League for Nursing, 1979.

The impact of technology on the practice of nursing has had multiple effects on the ethical relationship between nurse and patient. Prior to the miracle drugs and the rapid technological advances in medicine in this century, nursing and its caring functions were the main contributions to health care. The focus was on care of the hopelessly ill individual and not the instant cure of disease. As the practice of medicine became more enhanced in the cure of disease, the quantity and quality of caring on the part of nurses decreased and the nurse became an extension of the physician's technology. The nurse as a medical technician has led to a model of nursing care that is fragmented, dehumanized, and depersonalized. Loss of its caring identity and the abandonment of its caring functions has threatened the basic structure of nursing. A return to caring concern now offers hope for the future of nursing as nurses begin to value the types of caring services they are capable of rendering to those patients beyond the reach of medical technology—the chronically ill, the elderly, and the terminally ill.

The second major social force that has had a great impact on the ethical relationship between nurse and patient is the industrialization and subsequent bureaucratization of hospitals that began at the turn of the century. Alvin Toffler succinctly identifies three outstanding characteristics of a bureaucracy—performance, hierarchy, and a division of labor.[3] Performance is the recognition by the individual that she or he is dependent upon the institution and, hence, that her or his relationship to it will be an enduring one. Permanance necessarily brings about commitment by the individual to the organization and the more she or he invests her- or himself in the organization, the more her or his future becomes dependent on it. Realizing that she or he is dependent on the bureaucracy and that her or his future will be relatively permanent, the individual looks to the organizational hierarchy for approval and rewards and punishments. Subservience becomes conditioned over time and the powerful hierarchy through which the authority flows keeps the individual in line. The individual's actions are strictly defined by the rules of the organization, and the worker must carry out her or his specific task in the division of labor.

A growing body of historical research in nursing has revealed that as hospitals became more bureaucratic in structure they relied upon the nurse to further the goals of medical science and hospital administration. Ashley's very revealing study clearly shows how hospital administrators and physicians have controlled the educational and practice settings for the nurse and, hence, controlled the socialization process in nursing.[4] Let us look for a moment at the effects of these social forces on the values of nurses and the types of nurse–patient relationships that they have fostered. Based on data I have collected on the moral reasoning of nurses, I have found that, while the values of nurses do differ, a significant number of nurses are not oriented toward the rights and claims of patients when they are faced with ethical conflicts. Using hypothetical moral dilemmas, which presented conflicts between human needs or the welfare of others and adherence to the commands of authority or obedience to legal-social rules, I found three basic ways in which nurses viewed the nurse–patient relationship. The following models reflect the three types of orientation—the bureaucratic model, the physician advocate model, and the patient advocate model.[5]

Bureaucratic Model of the Nurse–Patient Relationship

In the bureaucratic model, the nurse is expected to focus on the details of coordinating institutional activities and she must not get involved with patients and their families because she might lose sight of her role and what is expected of her. The prescribed role of the nurse severely limits her responsibility and accountability to individual patients and the emphasis is on team work and team responsibility. Given the social structure of the health care system, the physician is the authority figure and gives the orders. The nurse has an "ethical obligation" to the physician and she does not have the right to go against him or her. The nurse must be fully aware of her limitations and she must not overstep the bounds of her prescribed role because it will disrupt team functioning. The patient is expected to forego individual rights, privileges, and freedoms for the greater good of all the other patients and health care personnel.

Role of Health Care Professionals in the Bureaucratic Model

The nurse is a buffer, catalyst, spokesperson, and police officer for the physician and hospital administration. She is expected to focus on the details of coordinating institutional activities and the enforcement of rules and regulations dictated by physicians and hospital administrators. The nurse must be able to define clearly her role in the institutional hierarchy and she must be aware of her limitations at all times. The physician is the head of the team and is ultimately responsible for the patient's care. The nurse is accountable to the physician and the people in higher positions in the bureaucratic system. Nursing emphasis is on team responsibility and accountability and not on individual patient responsibility or accountability.

Rights and Duties of Health Care Professionals in the Bureaucratic Model

The physician is the leader of the health care team by virtue of his or her education, expertise, and position of authority in the bureaucratic hierarchy. Rapport between members of the health care team takes priority over patients' needs because, if team members are opposed, the institution will not be able to function well. The nurse is expected to show respect for physician and administrative authority at all times. She must be concerned with maintaining loyalty to authority figures in the institutional system of order and must go through all the bureaucratic channels if conflict arises.

The nurse must not get involved with patients because she might lose sight of her role and what is expected of her. Socio-legal concerns and institutional policies determine the nature of nurses' communication with patients and their families. Since the nurse always carries out the physician's orders, it is not up to her to make decisions about the patient and she has no right to go against the physician's orders.

Role of the Patient in the Bureaucratic Model

The patient is expected to know his or her role in the health care system and must understand the limitations of the nurse's role as defined by the particular institution. The patient is perceived as an entity to be serviced by the health care system in a manner which allows the bureaucracy to carry out its functions in the most efficient and cost effective manner. As a passive and willing subject, the patient is expected to cooperate and make it possible for nurses and other health team members to function with a minimum of disturbance.

Rights and Duties of Patients in the Bureaucratic Model

Rights of the patient are defined by the institution and they may be restricted for the sake of social order and the welfare of the institution or health care team. The patient is expected to allow health care personnel to do things to him or her without questioning or resisting their authority and health care personnel can do anything they feel is in the best interest of the patient or institution. The patient has the right only to expect the nurse to perform within her prescribed role as dictated by the particular institution and the health care hierarchy. In the interests of maintaining a smoothly running institution and good team relationships, the patient is expected to accept the fact that the nurse must support her co-workers at all times when any moral conflict arises.

Goal of the Bureaucratic Model

The goal of the bureaucratic model is the maintenance of the social order and the smooth functioning of the health care institution. Patients are used to further the ends of the bureaucracy and can be used as means to achieve desired ends. Nurses focus on the technical or doing aspects of nursing and they keep interpersonal contact and communication with patients at a minimum in order to achieve the most efficient level of functioning for the institution.

Physician Advocate Model of the Nurse–Patient Relationship

In the second model, the physician advocate model, the nurse is viewed as an extension of the physician, operating in the medical model of science and technology. The nurse strives to enhance the authority of the physician and her duty is to instill in the patient confidence in the doctor. Whenever there is a question regarding the physician's treatment, the nurse is expected to defend the physician's decisions regardless of their rightness or wrongness. If the patient realized the physician's shortcomings, it could cause mistrust between physician and patient. Because the patient is only present for a short while, the physician's relationship with the nurse counts more than the patient's relationship, and the nurse must stay on the good side of the doctor. The patient and nurse are expected to trust the doctor at all times, because no matter what the doctor does he or she has a reason and means well. The goal of the physician advocate model is to maintain a trustful and harmonious relationship between nurse and physician as well as between physician and patient even if it is at the expense of the nurse–patient relationship.

Role of Health Care Professionals in the Physician Advocate Model

The nurse is an extension of the physician and therefore is expected to operate in the medical model of science and technology. She acts as a catalyst and interpreter in the doctor–patient relationship and mediates conflicts between physician, patients, and their families. In a conflict between patient and family and physician, the nurse is expected to value her relationship with the physician and to act on the physician's claims while ignoring those of the patient or family.

Rights and Duties of Health Care Professionals in the Physician Advocate Model

Since the nurse seeks harmonious, non-skeptical relationships with physicians, she must have the trust, respect, and cooperation of the doctor at all times. The nurse is expected to be loyal and to trust the physician's judgment and she must cover up any of the physician's errors. The nurse's duty is to instill in the patient trust and confidence in the physician and to maintain a good working relationship with the physician.

Role of the Patient in the Physician Advocate Model

The role of the patient is to understand that the nurse and doctor are trying to help her or him and that, therefore, she or he should cooperate and trust them to make all the decisions. The patient should try to maintain harmony between nurse and doctor and should not do anything that would threaten or interfere with the nurse–physician relationship.

Rights and Duties of Patients in the Physician Advocate Model

The patient is expected to cooperate fully with the physician since the latter has good reasons for making decisions and always means well. The patient is expected to understand that the nurse works hard and is under stress at some times, but that everything she does is for the good of the patient and physician. Since patients can be used to further the ends of medical science and technology, they are expected to comply with all therapy and research regimens that help to further the goals of the physician.

Goal of the Physician Advocate Model

The goal of the physician advocate model is the maintenance of a trustful and harmonious relationship between nurse and physician and between physician and patient. Patients can be used as means to achieve the desired end of a good nurse–physician relationship.

Patient Advocate Model of the Nurse–Patient Relationship

In the patient advocate model, the nurse considers her moral authority to be as great as any other health care professional and no one can command the nurse's morality or ethics. The nurse is seen as having a role of her own to carry out. She does not become part of the doctor–patient relationship and she is not subservient to medicine or hospital administration. Since the nurse spends so much more time with the patient and has a more continuous, caring relationship with the patient than any other member of the health care team does, she is able to develop a more insightful relationship with the patient. Hence the close, intense nature of the nurse–patient relationship often places the nurse in the best position to make decisions about the patient. The goal of the nurse is not to receive gratification from other health care professionals but rather to help the patient obtain the best possible care even if it means going against hospital administration and other health care professionals.

Role of Health Care Professionals in the Patient Advocate Model

The nature of the physician's authority over the nurse–patient relationship is irrelevant and the physician's authority is limited to the field of medicine. Nurses and physicians have equal responsibility for their own actions and the nurse is not an extension of the physician. Since the nurse's professional evaluation of the patient's needs and symptomatology is of equal value to the physician's, the nurse should be an equal contributor in the planning and implementation of the patient's care. The nurse's primary role is to act in the best interests of the patient and her accountability is to the patient, not to the physician or hospital administrator. Patients, families, and health care personnel are treated as equal, autonomous persons rather than in terms of their status and role in the health care system.

Rights and Duties of Health Care Professionals in the Patient Advocate Model

The nurse is obligated to respect the dignity and privacy of the patient as a person. Since all people are equal and have the same basic rights, no one health professional has any more rights than the patient or any other health professional. The nurse considers her moral authority to be as great as that of any other health care professional and she rejects the charismatic authority of the physician as "leader" of the health care team. An ideal nurse–physician relationship requires the recognition of each as a free and equal individual. Concern for what is right or fair, not obligations to or relationships with other health care personnel, determines the nurse's orientation to the patient. The nurse has primary responsibility to and accountability for the patient before the institution or other members of the health care team.

Role of the Patient in the Patient Advocate Model

The patient is expected to maximize his or her participation in all phases of his or her care. As an intelligent and informed consumer, the patient is responsible for his or her own life and the patient, not the health care professional, makes his or her own decisions. Since the patient has the right to receive the best possible care, he or she is not expected to allow him- or herself to be manipulated for the sake of medical science, the bureaucracy, or the gratification of health care personnel.

Rights and Duties of Patients in the Patient Advocate Model

The patient and family have the right to be treated with dignity and respect. The patient has a right to receive honest and accurate information about her or his illness so that she or he can make intelligent, informed decisions about her or his life. The patient has the right to question treatment or refuse certain aspects of it, since the extent of care given is determined by her or his needs and not the needs of other people.

Goal of the Patient Advocate Model

The goal of the model is the autonomy, self-actualization, and development of the patient as a unique individual. To achieve this, the nurse must act as an advocate for the patient in helping him or her to obtain whatever care is needed.

Since the values of nurses are expressed in these three models of the nurse–patient relationship, let us now look at how they affect the ethical decision making process in nursing. Nurses who operate in the physician advocate model are oriented toward maintaining harmonious relationships with physicians, authority figures, and institutions. They base their ethical decisions on approved solutions and they are guided by the "good intentions" and immediate wishes of authority figures.[6] The nurse who reasons in this manner has a conception of justice that is restricted to interpersonal relationships of family and significant others and cannot be extended beyond concrete, interpersonal relationships. If the nurse does not perceive the patient as a personal friend, there is little chance that the patient will be treated justly in all situations of moral conflict. In all likelihood, the nurse will perceive physicians, supervisors, and colleagues as significant others and will direct her attention toward their claims when moral conflict arises.

Nurses who operate in the bureaucratic model are guided by the rules of authority figures and institutional regulations, and, for them, justice becomes a principle for social order rather than for personal moral choice. Being unable to engage in moral reasoning that weighs competing claims of each individual in moral situations results in unthinking obedience that renders the nurse helpless when faced by conflicts of duty. Instead of functioning as a responsible moral agent when faced with decisions of principle that must do justice to the uniqueness of each situation, the nurse submits to the edict of superiors and the fixed rules and regulations of the institution.[7]

In terms of ethical theory, the bureaucratic and physician advocate models of the nurse–patient relationship lend themselves to what is referred to in moral philosophy as a consequentialist-utilitarian type of ethical decision. For the consequentialist-utilitarian an act is right if it is useful in bringing about the desirable end of maximizing good, pleasure, or happiness. The theory is concerned only with the consequences of actions and not with the means one chooses to achieve good ends. In making decisions one lists the available alternatives and assigns a value of good-evil, pleasure-pain, or happiness-unhappiness. After completion of the utilitarian calculus, the ethically correct choice is the alternative with the highest value of good, pleasure, or happiness.[8]

What, then, are the implications for this kind of utilitarian framework in nursing practice? Compared with the patient advocate model the bureaucratic and physician advocate models are obviously deficient in almost all their dimensions in terms of the human rights of the patient. When utilitarians assert that each person's good is to count equally, it means that whose good is affected by the act or rule is irrelevant to the calculation. The greatest total balance of pluses over minuses actually requires that one or more individuals sacrifice for the good of many. For the utilitarian, individual personal relationships with patients are not important. Utilitarians are concerned with the quantity, not quality, of relationships. You simply count up each relationship and sum them up in your calculus. In a temporal sense, the utilitarian framework is oriented toward current and future relationships. On-going or past relationships with patients are not important to the nurses' commitment, fidelity, or promise keeping. The theory's means-to-ends reasoning allows patients to be used as mere means, and can lead to morally unacceptable ends in terms of the individual patient's best interests.[9] The utilitarian framework in nursing lends itself to what philosopher Martin Buber has referred to as the I-It relationship where the patient becomes a thing to be manipulated or used as a means to further the needs of technology, medical science, and the health care bureaucracy.[10]

The utilitarian framework of ethical decision making in nursing that stems directly from the impact of social forces in this century has been the guiding force in our assembly line production nursing care. The norms of nursing action have been governed by the utilitarian calculus of cost-benefit analysis which is concerned with use of the least expensive means to bring about the ends or goals of the bureaucracy.[11] If the moral implications of the effect of cost-benefit analysis on the nurse–patient relationship had become apparent in the past, they would have created unmanageable conflict in nurses. In order to ward off such conflict, the bureaucratic and physician advocate models were conceived and imposed upon nursing, and nurses were socialized to focus on technical issues in the course of their daily labors. The "professional" nurse did not get involved with patients and she separated her feelings, emotions, and caring concerns from her "professional" self.

Nurses who operate in the bureaucratic model can easily be caught up in the guilt of what Hannah Arendt referred to as "bureaucratic violence." Whenever administrative or bureaucratic violence occurs, there is a vertical division of moral labor in institutions where the top administrative levels (hospital administrators and physicians) make all the important value decisions that determine goals and ends. The middle level administrators (nursing administration) are relegated to coordination or means decisions of technical efficacy, while the lowest level individuals (staff nurses) obey the orders unquestioningly, performing only one small aspect of labor. At these lower levels there is no accountability or moral responsibility for one's role in the larger action.[12] The nurses who operate in the bureaucratic or physician advocate model can only respond to moral situations with a pre-ordained, stereotypical response because they fail to recognize that alternatives exist. Since they do not choose freely or responsibly, they cannot be held accountable for their actions to the patient.

In opposition to the bureaucratic, physician advocate, utilitarian type of ethical decision making in nursing, the patient advocate model lends itself to the deontological or ethical formalist model of decision making. For the ethical formalist, an action is right if it is in accordance with a moral rule and it is wrong if it violates such a rule.[13] Moral rules are always based on an ultimate principle of duty and the test of rightness is not the badness or goodness of consequences. Concern is for the kind of action in question and whether or not it satisfies the supreme principle of duty to the Moral Law. In the Kantian tradition, the Moral Law is summarized in the categorical imperative to treat a person always as an end in her- or himself and never as a means only. Operating in this framework, a moral relationship among nurses and patients is one in which the patients' autonomy, dignity, and worth are respected, precluding using the patient as a mere means to the ends of medical science or the bureaucracy.

What then are the implications of an ethical formalist framework of ethical decision making for nursing practice? In keeping with the philosophy of the patient advocate model there is an emphasis on special relationships between nurse and patient in this model. Each nurse–patient relationship is unique and has inherent worth; the quality, not quantity, of relationships is of overriding importance to the nurse. The nurse's past relationship as well as her continuing and future relationships with patients are paramount. A human, caring, highly personal relationship exists and the nurse has a time perspective that incorporates past, present, and future actions. The nurse is oriented toward duty, responsibility, fidelity, and commitment to the patient when she is faced with conflict. Patients are not perceived as a mechanism to be worked upon but rather as conscious human beings with dignity and worth who are able to make choices and consequently can be free to do so.

Much lip service is given currently to the patient advocate model in health care, but if one looks at contemporary social forces in operation, the medical model of science and technology and the bureaucratic models of health care delivery prevail. There seems to be a huge gap between nursing's espoused theories and action. Our profession can follow the course it has been on, and merely go on complying with the social forces imposed upon it, or we can renew the spirit of the Nightingale era and we can become *the* social force that turns the health care system around.

The public is losing confidence in the health professional's ability to serve it in its own best interests. An ever increasing move on the part of society to have outside advocates and ombudsmen for patients clearly conveys the message that the public assumes nurses and patients are engaged in adversarial kinds of relationships. We must take careful stock of our values and we must begin to truly ask ourselves what really are the goals of nursing? Is it the smooth functioning of the bureaucracy? Is it the furtherance of medical science and technology or is it the best possible *care* for the patient? If we decide that our ends are the furtherance of the bureaucracy and medical technology, then we should keep right on with many of our current decisions and actions, because we have been, and still are, achieving those goals. If we determine that the end of nursing is the best possible care for patients then we must create new means to achieve this end.

If we are serious about our commitment to patients and we wish to make ethical decisions that take their best interests into account, we can begin to take a look at nursing's means to this end by heeding Paul Ramsey, philosopher and theologian. Ramsey holds that the ultimate and binding requirement for legitimate participation in the ethical decision making process on the part of the health care providers is in the capacity of their role as care givers not as cure givers.[14] For Ramsey, the basis of care becomes the source of our particular moral obligation and the court of final appeal for deciding the features of our practice that make what we do right or wrong. In the course of our caring, Ramsey maintains, we have to be concerned with two sorts of questions. First, when we are faced with an ethical dilemma, we must ask the question: Which of our actions in the situation take most *care* of human life? Second, he maintains, we must be concerned about the "rules of the game" in practice, and we must ask the question: What rules of practice will render actions that are most careful and respectful of the dignity of all concerned in the situation?

If we take Ramsey seriously and we begin to look at current nursing actions in particular situations and we examine our rules of practice, we are faced with the reality that nursing education and practice have got to change. As we look to the future, we must ask ourselves what kind of education is needed to adequately prepare the nurse to function as a patient advocate? Likewise, we must ask ourselves what kind of practice setting is needed to maintain our idealized nurse–patient relationship? How should nursing practice be organized and controlled? While I do not by any means propose to have all the answers, I would like to make some recommendations as they relate to nursing education and service settings.

The role of the humanities in the development of values and human insight has long been recognized. It has been acknowledged that the humanities impart appreciation of freedom, autonomy, individuality, and sensitivity in individuals. Ashley documented in her study how hospitals and physicians deliberately prevented nurses from being educated in the humanities because such exposure might create values that would be inconsistent with values needed to function in the bureaucratic structure of hospitals.[15] The virtues of subservience to, docility toward, and blind obedience of authority needed to function in institutions are hardly consistent with the appreciation of freedom, autonomy, and creativity gained from the humanities.

Nursing educators need to seriously examine the current relationship between nursing and the humanities in their curriculum. All too often, nursing's association with the humanities has been a fleeting one at best, and the baccalaureate student gets it out of the way in the first two years of her education so that she can then be educated to function in a technological environment. While students should be exposed to humanities courses at the beginning of their baccalaureate education, previous knowledge gained of the human condition must be integrated into clinical application at a later date when it is so badly needed to sensitize students to the plight of their patients.

The survival of nursing demands that we supply professionals adept in the ways of skills and machines, but humanistic insight cries for the sensitivity of fellowship in the human relationship that ensues in the performance of occupational duties. We need only acknowledge the notable success of a Nightingale or a Kübler-Ross to recognize that society looks for the reliable practitioner to interpret and appreciate the universals of the humanities while concurrently exercising flawless scientific skill. It is a given that society needs the ministering of the nurse on a purely physical basis. It is likely that, when that service is given in more conscious recognition of the diversity of patients as people, nursing will be recognized as the truly humane profession it claims to be in this time when the forces of technology seek to capture humanity's sensitive nature. So, physically, people need nursing to restore their well-being as functioning societal components. But people are not mere mechanical components, and the prospect of restoring them physically is dim if their more deeply human needs are not met as well as the "mechanics" of their physical needs.

In order to prepare nurses to function as moral agents, it is necessary to examine the socialization process in nursing to determine its effect on the values of nurses. We must create educational and service environments that foster moral commitment and autonomy. In addition to increased exposure to the broad humanities, students must gain expertise in ethical decision making. They must receive a foundation in ethical theory and they must be guided through the ethical decision making process as they encounter actual dilemmas in clinical practice.

Moral development theory and research holds that ethical reasoning and development progress from a preconventional level in childhood, where the individual responds to external rules according to physical or pleasure-seeking consequences, to a conventional level in adolescence, where the individual is oriented toward maintaining expecations of significant others or the larger society.[16] At this conventional level, concern is directed toward maintaining, supporting, and justifying the social order. At the postconventional or autonomous level of morality, the individual attempts to define moral values and principles that have application and validity separate from group norms and authority. Autonomous, postconventional, principled morality is achieved in adulthood and it is only when one is in the mid to late twenties that one is capable of acting in an autonomous moral way when faced with conflict. One of the critical periods of development occurs late in adolescence and the college years when a student is more open and responsive to environmental stimulation.

Research findings to date on moral development have stressed the importance of considering the individual in relation to the moral environment or atmosphere in which she or he functions. Studies that have looked at the moral atmosphere in educational settings confirm that students respond best to a combination of moral reasoning, moral action, and the institutional rules as a unified whole in relation to the manner in which they make moral judgments. The potential of a moral atmosphere to foster autonomous moral reasoning depends upon a high level of justice that is based on democracy and fairness and recognizes the dignity and self worth of the learner or practitioner. Moral commitment and responsibility are fostered in environments that allow individuals to partake in the decision making process. The more the individual shares in decision making, the more she or he is able to take on the moral perspective of other people and the more she or he becomes actively involved in the social and moral functioning of the school and practice environment. A number of studies in nursing practice settings have shown how the social organization of the health care institution affected the value orientation and role performance of the nurse.[17]

In studying the organizational structure of a large mental hospital and its effect on patterns of patient care, the Bueker study found that on units where authoritarian systems of organization prevailed the following effects were noted:

1. The supervisory staff were punitive, authoritarian, and status conscious, and there was an emphasis on maintaining power and adherence to a rigid, formal structure.
2. There was resentment, insecurity, and distrust among the staff.
3. Staff were alienated from their values and roles and they were reluctant to assume responsibility. Nurses were submissive to medical power and their values focused on meeting their own utilitarian needs.
4. There was a non-humanistic perception of patients and they were regarded as inferior beings with limited rights and extensive obligations.
5. There was an absence of therapeutic programs and no evidence of therapeutically structured nurse–patient or doctor–patient interaction.
6. There were neglectful patterns of patient care and evidence of patient abuse and whatever care existed was custodial, task-oriented, and impersonal in nature.

In contrast, on the units where the democratic, consultative, and more patient-centered system of organization prevailed, the following conditions were found to be in existence:

1. Supervisory and medical staff were democratic and understanding and treated the staff with respect. The competencies of supervisors and staff were equated not with their ascribed status in the organization but with their demonstrated abilities.
2. The basic philosophy of the unit was egalitarian and emphasized shared responsiblity, collaboration, group decision making, and control.
3. There was an open system of communication and staff were warm, mutually supportive, and goal-oriented.
4. The hospital was viewed as an environment that could be manipulated for fostering the personal growth of individuals and it was adapted to fit the needs of patients.
5. The treatment milieu was very patient-centered and therapeutically oriented. There was a high degree of staff-patient interaction and humanistic perceptions of patients, and there was a regard for the patient as a person who had dignity and rights to participate in her or his own care.

Nursing educators must create an atmosphere of mutual trust, respect, and openness so that there can be honest dialogue between teacher and student and they must encourage moral reflection that involves identity questioning and consistency between moral reasoning and action. Nursing students must be exposed to moral discourse that presents moral conflict and contradiction to their current moral thinking structures in order to create states of cognitive disequilibrium that lead to moral growth and further development.[18] In nursing practice, environments that allow nurses to act as moral agents for their patients must be created. Since the traditional role of the nurse has been one of subservience and unquestioning loyalty and obedience to authority, it stands to reason that the bureaucratic and physician advocate models of moral reasoning are functional for the role that the nurse has been forced to play in the health care system.

Kramer's extensive research has found that baccalaureate graduates change from a professional value orientation to a bureaucratic value orientation after they have been in the work setting following their graduation.[19] In light of a theory of moral development, they are in all likelihood at a stage of moral development where they conform to the role stereotype as conceived by the educational setting and, because the service setting offers no more than a bureaucratic moral atmosphere, they become arrested at that stage of moral development. The young graduate is at a critical period of ethical development and instead of expecting her to be an initiator of social change, we should be exposing her to a moral atmosphere that fosters and supports autonomous moral action on behalf of patients. Mere cognitive awareness of universal moral principles must be developed into a commitment to their application in the ethical practice of nursing.

Nursing must also take stock of the present models of delivery of nursing practice in institutional settings. In many understaffed institutions, nurses are forced to practice triage in the allocation of a scarce resource, namely their nursing care. Again we must raise the question what are the ends and means relationships in the goals of nursing? Is our goal to give the best possible care to one or a few patients at the cost of care to many patients or is it to give minimum, substandard care to as many patients as possible? If a nurse has a special relationship with a particular patient, no physician, institution, or other patient with greater needs should be able to demand that the nurse compromise her care for a patient to meet their needs.

Charles Fried, a lawyer and philosopher, observes that the ideal of professional loyalty to the lawyer's client demands an allocation of the lawyer's time and resources in ways that are not maximally conducive to the greatest good for the greatest number in society.[20] He points out that society always sanctions our acting partially toward those individuals who stand closest to us, such as those people with whom we hold a special relationship as in friendship or kinship, as opposed to the more abstract interests of humanity at large. Just as cost-benefit analyses in determining best possible consequences usually do not enter into decisions about friends or relatives, so too they should not enter into the nurse's decisions about a patient's welfare. We should establish rules of practice and models of nursing practice such that the nurse is morally obligated to adopt as her goal the furthering of the patient's interests above the collective interest. The nurse's primary loyalty should be to the individual patient whatever his or her situation or need.

The present-day identity crisis of women as members of society and as members of the nursing profession, the realization that nursing's recent value system has been inadequate, and the opportunity for nurses to assume increased moral responsibility for the welfare of their patients are the hallmarks necessary for stimulation of nurses to autonomous moral reasoning. The profession of nursing now has the potential to achieve a new level of moral development—one at which we define our moral values and principles separate from bureaucratic norms and authority.

Endnotes

1. For a further analysis see "The Moral Situation in Nursing," by Catherine P. Murphy in *Bioethics and Human Rights: A Reader for Health Professionals,* ed. Elsie L. Bandman and Bertram Bandman (Boston: Little, Brown, 1978), pp. 313–320; and Catherine P. Murphy, "Levels of Moral Reasoning in a Selected Group of Nursing Practitioners," (Ed.D. dissertation, Teachers College, Columbia University, 1976).
2. Josephine A. Dolan, *Nursing in Society: A Historical Perspective* (Philadelphia: W. B. Saunders, 1978), pp. 43–85.
3. Alvin Toffler, *Future Shock* (New York: Random House, 1970), pp. 144–145.
4. Jo Ann Ashley, *Hospitals, Paternalism and the Role of the Nurse* (New York: Teachers College Press, 1976).
5. I am greatly indebted to Lawrence Kohlberg, Daniel Candee, and the staff of the Harvard University Moral Education Research Foundation for the formulation of many of my ideas and research in this area. Kohlberg's theory and scoring system for analysis of moral reasoning enabled me to develop a framework for these models of the nurse-patient relationship.
6. For a more complete discussion of this type of moral reasoning see N. Haan, M. Brewster Smith, and Jeanne Block "Moral Reasoning of Young Adults: Political-Social Behavior, Family Background, and Personality Correlates," *Journal of Personality and Social Psychology* 10, no. 3 (1968), pp. 183–201.
7. Further discussion of this type of moral reasoning can be found in Lawrence Kohlberg "From Is to Ought: How to Commit the Naturalistic Fallacy and Get Away with it in the Study of Moral Development," in *Cognitive Development and Epistemology,* ed. T. Mischel (New York: Academic

Press, 1971); and A. I. Melden "Moral Education and Moral Action," in *Moral Education Interdisciplinary Approaches,* ed. Clive M. Beck, Brian S. Critten, and Edmund V. Sullivan (Toronto: University of Toronto Press, 1971).

8. Paul W. Taylor, *Principles of Ethics: An Introduction* (Encino, Calif.: Dickenson Publishing, 1975), pp. 55–81.

9. I wish to acknowlege the contribution of James F. Childress, former Joseph P. Kennedy Sr. Professor of Christian Ethics at the Kennedy Institute, in helping me to formulate these ideas during the course of my participation in the National Endowment for the Humanities Seminar on Ethical Issues in Health Care Delivery at Georgetown University in the summer of 1978.

10. Martin Buber, *I and Thou,* trans. Walter Kaufman (New York: Charles Scribner's Sons, 1970).

11. Alasdair MacIntyre, "Utilitarianism and Cost-Benefit Analysis: An Essay on the Relevance of Moral Philosophy to Bureaucratic Theory" in *Values in the Electric Power Industry,* ed. C. K. Sayre (Notre Dame, Indiana: University of Notre Dame Press, 1977), pp. 217–237.

12. For a more complete discussion of this topic see Lawrence Kohlberg and Peter Scharf "Bureaucratic Violence and Conventional Moral Thinking," *American Journal of Ortho Psychiatry,* (April 1972).

13. Taylor, *Principles of Ethics,* pp. 82–113.

14. Paul Ramsey, "Conceptual Foundations for an Ethics of Medical Care: A Response" in *Ethics and Health Policy,* ed. Robert M. Veatch and Roy Branson (Cambridge, Mass.: Ballinger, 1976), pp. 48–49.

15. Ashley, *Hospitals, Paternalism and the Role of the Nurse,* pp. 16–33.

16. Kohlberg, "From Is to Ought."

17. Kathleen Bueker, "A Study of the Social Organization of a Large Mental Hospital" (Ph.D. dissertation, The American University, 1969). H. Harrington and E. Theis, "Institutional Factors Perceived by Baccalaureate Graduates as Influencing their Performances as Staff Nurses," *Nursing Research* 17 (1968), pp. 228–235. V. Jarett, "A Study of Conceptions of Autonomous Nursing Actions Appropriate for the Staff Nurse Role" (Ph.D. dissertation, University of Texas, 1967). Laura Simms, "The Hospital Staff Nurse Position as Viewed by Baccalaureate Graduates in Nursing" (Ph.D. dissertation, Teachers College, Columbia University, 1963).

18. Murphy, "The Moral Situation in Nursing," pp. 317–320.

19. Marlene Kramer, *Reality Shock: Why Nurses Leave Nursing* (St. Louis: C. V. Mosby, 1974).

20. Charles Fried, "The Lawyer as Friend: The Moral Foundations of the Lawyer–Client Relation," *Yale Law Journal* 85, no. 8 (July 1976), pp. 1060–1089.

The conditions under which nurses practice today are increasingly dominated by circumstances which tend to depersonalize the relationship between the nurse and the patient. We have only to think of the impersonality of the computer-based operations by which we enter the hospital and the vast array of technological devices by which we are surrounded in the hospital to remember that health care is no longer conducted as it used to be. When the pressures to become a cog in a vast bureaucratic organization or to become as much a tender of machines as of persons are practically irresistible, it is crucial that the nurse never forget her original high calling as a member of a humane profession.

The essay by Howard Hunter offers an interpretation of nursing as a profession whose proper characteristics are those of the humane arts. He argues that there is a very real sense in which nurses have to be ministers, philosophers, and psychologists. Nurses have a unique opportunity—and an obligation—to provide the profoundly personal dimension in health care. Accordingly, they have to recognize that to be able to provide the quality of care demanded requires the development of personal qualities and skills in the area of the humanities.

2

Nursing: A Humane Profession

Howard Hunter

I was handed the phone when I entered the house. "It's for you. It's about your mother. She and Mrs. Miller have been in an accident." I took the phone—it was more than three years ago but it seems like yesterday—and was informed that my mother and her companion had been struck by a large truck while driving. I was urged to take the next plane home at once. I did so and thus began days of anxious waiting in a little room adjacent to the Intensive Care Unit in a mid-western hospital. Attached to an impressive array of complicated machinery, my mother and her companion were being sustained. Mercifully enough for her, my mother's companion died after a few days on the machines. Her injuries were sufficient to have left her in a permanently vegetative state had the doctors been successful in keeping her technically alive. My mother rallied, and now, more than three years after the accident, is still confined to the complete care area of a nursing home.

I shall never forget how difficult it was to secure helpful and thorough information about my mother's condition and her prognosis from the doctors in the hospital. Each appeared to be an effective technician. Each was a competent specialist. There was a doctor for my mother's lungs. There was a doctor for her bones. There was a doctor for her internal organs. There was a doctor for her heart. She was fortunate. But where, I began to ask myself, was the doctor for my mother? Where was the person who knew her as the unique individual she is? Where was the person who took time to listen to her and not just to her lungs? Where was the doctor who would listen to her wishes regarding her own health and treatment? I was eager to speak with the health care provider who knew and cared about my mother as a person and not simply as an organic problem to be solved.

I recall vividly my attempt to personalize my one conversation with one of the specialists whom I literally blocked in the hall as he was rushing off presumably to another problem. I pointed toward the unit where my mother and her companion lay surrounded by the various monitoring devices and life-support systems to which they were attached and I said, "It's interesting to be in this situation. I teach a course in which we consider moral and ethical issues involved in heroic measures for treating accident and terminal illness cases." At once, the specialist's attitude stiffened. He said abruptly, "I do not see any such problem of heroic measures here," and he turned away and left. I never saw him again.

Should the reader wonder by this point what this account of a personal experience has to do with the subject of this book on ethical issues of the nurse–patient relationship, I hasten to say that I have deliberately chosen an intensely personal event because I believe it illustrates that health crises are always deeply personal. It illustrates also a fundamental difference between the way humanists and scientists go about their work. I am a humanist and both by precept and example I wish to stress here the humanistic dimension of health care issues. A person operating in the scientific mode is required to rule out the subjective dimensions of human experience. The humanist is required not to neglect them. I see nurses as the humanists of the health care profession and this paper will show why.

Returning to the story of my mother's accident and the treatment she received, I am happy to report that I did find persons caring for my mother who admirably filled and continue to fill the role I had unthinkingly expected medical specialists to be filling. These people were and are her nurses. It was the nurses who, more than any others, became involved with the whole person—both the physical body and the personality—of my mother. Three years later, it is still the nurses who know her condition most intimately. It is they who can and do give her family the clearest explanations of her condition. It is they who are most available and accessible. It is they who minister to her and who most affect the very quality of her day-to-day and hour-to-hour life. While the medical specialists were admirably effective in meeting certain physical crises at a particular time of trauma, it is the nurses who provide the consistent long-term health care. Medical intervention for her, as for all of us, is actually an episode within the larger drama of health care in which the major actors are the nurses.

The quality of the health care the nurses provide my mother is measured, in the final analysis, not by their effectiveness in doing routine chores nor by their technical skills—as important and necessary as such skills are. Rather, the effectiveness of the nurses depends on their effectiveness as *persons*. There is a very real sense in which the nurses have to be ministers and philosophers and psychologists. They have to understand that a human being is more than a collection of organs. They have to demonstrate their care for persons in need and they have to do it wisely. They need to love wisdom, to have wisdom, to impart wisdom. They need to see what is of greatest value in one's life and they need to be able to communicate their insights to persons who are in need. It is part of the nurses' actual job, whether it appears in the job description or not, to be extraordinarily sensitive humanists who are able and willing to apply their humane competence in very specific and often very difficult circumstances.

Occasionally, when I have discussed my ideas about medical specialists and nurses with members of the medical and nursing professions, I have been given a somewhat cynical rejoinder which goes like this: "That business about doctors and nurses needing to be philosophers and ministers sounds good, but, let's face it, would you want a philosopher to take out your appendix?" After reflecting on that question for some time, I have concluded that in a very real sense I do want a philosopher for my doctor and for my nurse. Obviously, I do not want only a philosopher, but I want a doctor or a nurse who is also a philosopher. I want a doctor who has "philosophized" about the issues of life which go beyond the organ or systems of his or her own narrow specialty. I want a nurse who has cultivated the gifts of her own intelligence and her own spirit so that she has both the desire and the competence to work not only efficiently but wisely, humanely, with her patients. I want a nurse for whom courses in the humanities were something more than an obstacle to be "gotten out of the way" in a few perfunctory courses early in a program of nursing education.

I want a nurse who has resisted those forces within her training and her profession which have the effect—if not the intention—of making her an obedient bureaucrat, a technician, or a defender of someone's interests other than my own. I agree with nursing educator Dr. Jo Ann Ashley when she notes that some physicians and hospital administrators "fail to see much of a relationship between the quality of care received by patients and the education of the nurse."[1] Based on the personal experience I have presented here, an experience which is extremely common, I see the importance of nursing as a crucial factor in health care. Yet, as Dr. Ashley points out, "The importance of quality nursing is frequently not even mentioned in discussions on health care."[2] She urges us to see that an understanding of nurses and nursing is essential if we are to understand the crises, the defects, the needs, and the opportunities of today's health care systems. It is to such an understanding that this paper is addressed.

The primary assumption of this article is that nursing is or ought to be a humane profession. This simply means that nurses see or should see themselves as responsible individuals who are trying to achieve as full a development as possible of their own as well as others' personal maturity and authenticity. Nurses, like all other human beings, aspire or ought to aspire to become mature and fully realized human persons. At first glance, these statements seem so obvious as to be quite unnecessary. But that nursing is or should be a humane profession needs to be said for two very fundamental reasons. The first is that in actual practice nursing may turn out to be something other than primarily humane. It may, as a matter of fact, turn out to be something other than a professional activity if by profession we mean autonomy and self-determination. Nursing may turn out to be bureaucratic in that the nurse's duties are oriented more toward the goals of the institution employing her than to her patients. Nursing may turn out to be technical in that nursing practice becomes a matter of tending machines more than tending patients. It may turn out to be something other than a humane profession when the nurse's primary obligations are to her institution, to the medical profession, or to anything other than the patient she is called to serve. Nursing as a humane profession may be taken for granted as an ideal even in these situations, but as a practical matter it remains a goal very difficult, if not impossible, to realize. In fact, in such situations it may be a goal very difficult even to remember!

We need to remind ourselves that nursing is a humane profession for a second reason. It is very easy to say that nursing should be humane, but what does it mean to be humane? To act in a humane way requires that we know what this means and how to achieve it. But to be humane is not something that is realized simply with the announcement that one intends it. To be humane is a project requiring disciplined investigation, research, definitions, and constant scrutiny. It is much easier to state the desirability of being humane than it is to make certain that one has achieved the goal.

Seeing nursing as a humane profession provides a perspective from which to view and to evaluate the various situations and relationships in which the nurse finds herself. From this perspective nurses are obliged to ask themselves such questions as these: do the conditions of my preparation for nursing and my actual nursing practice support or do they prevent the achievement of a mature humaneness for me and for my patients? Within my profession is it possible for me to realize personal authenticity and to assist others to do the same? Does my professional situation allow for the development of genuinely moral activity? For activity to be moral there has to be the opportunity for choosing between alternatives. A moral situation requires that there be opportunities to consider alternative procedures and that the nurse determine the one most appropriate for her goals. Wherever the situation is one in which such freedom is absent, one has something other than a moral situation. In my nursing situation, am I given the opportunity for my own moral development?

With the perspective of nursing as a moral and humane profession—and one cannot be humane without having the opportunity to be moral—we see that every aspect of the nursing profession is a proper subject for serious scrutiny. The nurse's education, her practice, her relationships with patients, medical specialists, hospital staff, and administrators, families of patients, and the larger community all are subjects for critical examination. If any one aspect of the nurse's total context is lacking in significant dimensions of the moral and the humane, then the nurse's situation will itself be negatively affected, and both she and her patient will bear the burden.

It might well be asked: why is this matter of the humane and the moral a special problem for nursing? The answer, of course, is that it is not. The same task faces each individual in whatever circumstance she or he finds her- or himself. But recognizing the general nature of the obligation does not in any way reduce the necessity for the individual to confront the specific problems within a given profession. There are, however, at least five reasons, in addition to the general necessity just cited, nurses should recognize their obligation to be concerned with the definition and achievement of the humane within their profession.

First, the focus of the nurse's work is on the care of individuals whose own sense of personal wholeness, dignity, and health is in jeopardy through some form of mental or physical distress. The nurse is a member of the health care professions. She is regularly involved with persons undergoing personal crises regarding their own sense of well-being. The nurse must relate to persons whose experience is traumatic to them. As Dr. Sally Gadow reminds us elsewhere in this book, for the patient it is his or her whole self, not just his or her body as an object, that seeks attention and treatment. The nurse is required to develop a basic understanding of the dimensions of health which go beyond the physical condition of the body.

The nurse must have reflected on the meaning of health and of sickness. She must have considered the various interpretations placed on sickness within the several religions and cultures from which her patients are likely to come. What, she must ask herself, is the place of sickness in the scheme of things? Is it an enemy to be battled? a devil to be exorcised? an expression of a moral fault of which the patient is guilty? Is it an accident having no significance or is it a part of a divine plan? What is her attitude toward those who hold one or another of these views about sickness? Is terminal illness always to be combatted, always a tragedy?

In nursing situations where there is a high incidence of incurable illness and death, the high rate of staff turnover is very well documented. Is this due to the fact that terminal illness is itself somehow more repellent than other illnesses? This is hardly true. Rather, it is due to the fact that health care attendants have not themselves developed an adequate comprehension of their own and their patients' problems in confronting acute or chronic trauma and terminal illness. A philosophy of terminal illness and death is required for each person who seeks to live a humane, mature, and authentic existence.

Second, there is throughout the health care professions a sense of crisis. The career of every present and future nurse is affected. The word "crisis" refers to the act of making decisions and connotes, as well, a sense of urgency. The current situation in the health care field requires the making of decisions whose urgency is compelling for those involved in it. To do more than to offer a representative list of crisis situations requires more space than is available here. A crisis of confidence within health care exists regarding the ability of the professions to continue adequately to fulfill their obligations within existing structures. The headlines of newspapers across the country cite debates at the national level on financing of health care for the nation, while at the local level articles exposing the latest incompetence, greed, and inadequate service are common-place.

There is, unmistakably, a crisis of credibility regarding the health care professions by a public increasingly critical and demanding of improvement. Other crises relate to the necessity of making urgent ethical decisions in the area of nursing and the dilemmas of terminal illness and care for the dying, the right of the patient to accept or reject treatment, and the nature of the nurse–patient relationship. A crisis within the nursing profession relates to the vexing matter of conflicting loyalties of the nurse: Is the nurse responsible to the hospital, the patient, the physician, the patient's family, the state, herself? How shall the nurse meet the crises presented in the cases involving euthanasia, abortion, allocation of scarce medical resources, drugs, and behavior control? It is difficult for today's nurse to avoid these crisis situations, each of which has direct bearing on the humane dimensions of her profession.

Third, there is a tide of rising expectations and raised consciousness among all peoples and especially among minorities and the oppressed. Nursing, traditionally and still today a profession almost totally made up of women, has been affected by many attitudes of male-dominated societies. It is perhaps too much to say that the increase in the consciousness of women regarding the explicit and implicit sexism in contemporary American social structures and attitudes presents a crisis for the nursing profession as a whole. It appears at least to this observer that the profession of nursing is something of a sleeping giant in this regard. But, surely, for individual nurses the tensions between rising feminist expectations and the traditional and stereotyped patterns of nursing practice present significant crises. Who can begin to count the cost of sexism within the profession of nursing? And who can estimate the cost to the profession of the loss to it of countless able men and women who have either not thought of nursing as a profession because they assumed it was for women only or who rejected it for the same reason? As painful as it may be, one may hope that throughout the profession there will be increasing awareness of unanalyzed sexist assumptions with a resulting "crisis" which will bring about desirable changes.

Fourth, the society in which today's nurse works, especially in the United States, is extraordinarily complex. It forces individuals to make decisions rather than to be content with conventional or traditional views. Ours is a pluralist society. This means that it has within it a great number and variety of cultures and subcultures. It means that persons coming to maturity and practicing a career in this nation must come to terms with persons of many different backgrounds, beliefs, and values. It means that the United States is not a homogeneous culture. In some countries foreigners stand out. Here it is impossible, especially in the urban centers, to identify anyone as a foreigner. There is a great diversity of perspective, commitment, and aspiration among the peoples of the United States. For example, in a community in which I worked in New England for some years there were eleven distinct and recognizable ethnic groups within a small city of fewer than one hundred thousand persons.

Fundamental philosophical questions are forced upon all individuals living in such a cultural cauldron. Who am I? What should I do? How should I live my life? What is true? What is the meaning, if there is one, of life? Today's nurse in such a situation is the inheritor of, and, reluctantly or otherwise, a participant in a continuous reassessment of values. Constant confrontation by the challenge to conventional and traditional attitudes and practices produces almost intolerable pressures for many people. One often sees the results of such pressures in mental and physical illness. And these varieties of outlooks and styles of life become especially evident during the crises of mental and physical health.

Fifth, there is yet another challenge to conventional perspectives which touches upon the education for and practice of nursing quite specifically and which produces a basic crisis situation. That is the domination of the scientific outlook and the related increase in the use of technologically sophisticated machines in the health care fields. Science and technology are not identical, of course, but they have together presented contemporary society with an unavoidable crisis: the crisis of human and machine. The question is whether people shall control their inventions or be controlled by them.

This crisis leads inevitably toward an even deeper crisis: the crisis of faith. In attempting to resolve the crisis of human and machine one is forced to reflect upon human nature and destiny. These are matters in which religious faith plays an important role. It appears that people are gaining final control of their lives and world—their knowledge of the origins of life, their ability to reproduce it, and their capacity to destroy it are unparalleled. Can one continue to accept uncritically the traditional teaching of religion and society? Many persons have responded to these crises by reaffirming traditional perspectives as revelation, or by reinterpreting them as significant myths, or, not infrequently, by attempting to dismiss them altogether as either irrelevant, antiquated, or too complex to be useful.

It may seem to some that the crisis of faith is not especially relevant to the subject of moral issues in the nurse–patient relationship. Nothing, in fact, could be more relevant. Among health care providers, it is only the nurse who has the opportunity to treat her patient in a holistic manner. This simply means that she has the occasion to relate to the whole person being treated. She cannot do this well if she does not have a sufficient basic self-understanding as well as an understanding of her patient in her or his total situation, physical, mental, and spiritual. As nursing educator Dr. Carol Soares demonstrates in her excellent essay comparing nursing and medical diagnoses, it is the nurse whose diagnoses move beyond those of medicine. Medical diagnoses define pathological states of the physical organism of the patient. Nursing diagnoses define altered states of human functioning at not only the apparent physical level but also at the levels of consciousness. Medicine rests at the biophysical level, while nursing considers not only that level but the psychosocial, the cognitive-perceptual, and cultural-spiritual levels as well.

Soares shows how the biophysical system is vital in sustaining life, while the psychosocial system sustains the patient in his or her individuality and in his or her community. The cognitive-perceptual system assists the patient in sustaining and creating meaning in his or her everyday life. The cultural-spiritual level affords the patient the means to sustain meaning and purpose not only in the experienced but the as-yet-to-be-experienced world as well. Medicine's diagnoses are disease-oriented while nursing's diagnoses are person-oriented. Nursing diagnoses have not received the intensive and sustained research and publication they deserve. Soares rightly concludes that every professional practitioner has the responsibility "to examine and to critically evaluate his or her practice and, in this way, participate in the articulation and the rationalization of nursing practice."[3]

For the nurse to do effective diagnostic work at the levels Professor Soares describes requires that the student preparing for a nursing career have both intensive and extensive involvement in the academic fields known as the humanities. The humanities have been variously defined. They include at least the classics, as at Oxford. At most they are those studies enumerated by the American Council of Learned Societies in its identification of the humanities with "philosophy (including philosophy of law and philosophy of science), aesthetics, philology, languages, literature, and linguistics, archaeology, art history, musicology, history (including history of science, history of law, and history of religions), cultural anthropology, and folklore."[4] It does not matter that some persons in these fields would not see themselves as humanists. The point here is that nurses whose task involves dealing with total individuals cannot neglect the concerns that these disciplines reflect. A nurse may feel that she does not have the slightest interest in, say, religion. But she cannot deal adequately with her patient if she does not have an adequate understanding of the place religion plays in the patient's life. She herself may not feel that art is important to her life. But she ought not to fail to see that art has had a very great deal to do with the shaping of the culture in which she and her patients live.

Every nurse needs the critical perspective that studies in the humanities can provide. Humanities may claim to be the means by which truth and culture are made available to societies. Whether they are or not, the humanities are disciplines which require that their students become critical about all truth claims and all cultural values. To study the humanities means that one learns that the world we see is seen from our particular perspective. The study of the humanities helps the student move from naive realism, the unanalyzed assumption that the particular point of view we have is the definitive, the final view on the subject at hand. When one is presented with only one viewpoint about the world, for example, it is easy uncritically to assume the truth of the view presented and to regard those with other perspectives as mistaken and even immoral.

W. T. Jones has said that a goal of education should be to help students not merely to tolerate but to *enjoy* cognitive dissonance, cognitive ambiguity. He acknowledges that the current educational systems are good in teaching students to master specific trades and to develop skills for the professions. But he insists that the best education is that which assists students to step outside the prevailing system's confines. Today, the prevailing educational paradigm or world view is that of the sciences. Jones is right when he says that the humanities offer a necessary alternative.[5]

The humanities have much to offer to the nurse preparing for her professional duties. Dr. Sally Gadow has discussed two basic ways of thinking about the relationship between nursing and the study of the humanities.[6] One way, she notes, starts from the humanities disciplines with their various historical, aesthetic, and philosophical approaches to understanding human experience, and attempts to relate them to the practice of nursing. A second way, the one Dr. Gadow recommends, takes the nursing experience as the starting point and asks which of the humanities disciplines appear best suited to be of assistance in drawing the clearer picture of nursing and its special characteristics.

Dr. Gadow considers perplexing and important issues relating to the nurse's position in connection with her basic professional relationships. With reference to the nurse's relationship to her patient she asks that nursing education pay greater attention to the understanding of the human body, to the meaning of suffering, and to the problems caused by an ever-increasing involvement of technological apparatus in nursing. She asks whether there are any ethical problems unique to the nurse–patient relationship and suggests the importance of more analysis of this question. Noting that the nurse has an obligation to refuse an order which she sees as medically unsafe or unsound, she asks whether such an obligation exists regarding orders she may consider ethically indefensible. She sees the need to bring the disciplines of history, law, and moral philosophy to the ongoing discussion between nurses and other health care providers. She notes that the humanities afford opportunity for the nurse to become acquainted with the various images of the nurse which have appeared in various cultures. She encourages the nursing education establishment to include consideration of the images of the nurse and nursing as shown in the visual arts and in literature.

The image the nurse has of herself and her profession will largely determine the quality of her performance and will color every aspect of her relationship to her patients and to her community. If the nurse is presented with models throughout her education which are primarily bureaucratic and technical, then her career activities will reflect such an orientation. If the models are humanistic, she will reflect humanistic concerns within her professional activity. The concern of the present writer is that the nurse see herself as occupying a position requiring the greatest of sensitivities to other individuals.

The nurse is preeminently the humanist in health care today. It is she who has the most sustained, the most intimate, and the most influential relationship to the patient. She has the moral responsibility to speak out wherever she sees practices that have the actual (whether intended or not) effect of dehumanizing and depersonalizing individuals. The nurse does well to remember Mahatma Ghandi's response when asked what he considered the single greatest sin which human beings commit. He replied, "The hardness of heart of the educated classes." The nurse is simply not adequately prepared for her task who has not acknowledged the primary place of sensitivity and caring within the nursing profession.

Today's nurses are required to practice in an environment in which strong images available to previous generations are no longer so readily accessible to many. This point was demonstrated in a novel way to a number of my students through an exercise in connection with the following passage from a novel by André Malraux:

> The greatest mystery is not that we have been flung at random among the profusion of the earth and the galaxy of the stars, but that in this prison we can fashion images sufficiently powerful to deny our nothingness.[7]

We asked persons at several educational levels as well as mature adult individuals to sketch their interpretation of the passage. Nearly all the persons responding portrayed quite clearly the prison in one way or another, but very, very few either chose to or were able to portray a strong self-image. Also, quite revealingly, no one in any group questioned the idea that life is a prison and that our individual lives are nothing.

We can see in the unquestioning acceptance of this view of life the extent of the absence of traditional religious views. This modest exercise underscored the fact that today's nurses are treating persons who may very well be unusually vulnerable to those who promise what an attractive and viable image of personal authenticity provides. The nurse may easily find her patient placing too much trust in the nurse's words. One has only to think today of the vulnerability of distressed and disenfranchised persons such as those who played out the last dramas of their lives in the jungles of Guyana, destroying their bodies with the assurance that they were doing a spiritually significant deed.

The crisis of faith with which today's nurse is confronted is obviously too large a topic to discuss here. We can only note that it exists and that it presents nurses with some very specific necessities, opportunities, and challenges. This crisis of faith has been developing for a very long time and will not be eliminated in the lifetime of anyone living today. In a general way, there has been a crisis of faith ever since the moment a person first entertained a doubt about a prevailing opinion. But more specifically for our culture and our historical epoch, the crisis of faith may be seen to have its roots in the words of such figures as Copernicus, Darwin, Marx, and Freud and their intellectual descendents.

Once it was a matter of common faith—an unanalyzed assumption—that God had created a universe in which the world was the center. But the theories of Copernicus challenged this view. Today it is again taken for granted—an unanalyzed assumption for many—that no God created the universe, and, in any event, the world we know is not the center of the universe we have discovered. This new conviction—and it is precisely that for most persons who merely accept what scientists say today with as much credulity as their ancestors accepted what holy men said—required a change in the view humanity had of itself within creation.

Similarly, it was not very long ago, historically speaking, that it was commonly accepted that people were a special creation of God. But with the teaching of Charles Darwin and his followers regarding the evolution of humanity, this idea received a challenge of the most profound sort. Today Darwinian theory is taken for granted and the image of humanity has again had to undergo a significant change. It is commonplace for individuals in our culture no longer to see themselves as a special and unique creation of God but rather as a part of an evolutionary process.

The idea that people can be in control of their environment even though they are a part of evolutionary process came under attack with the work of Karl Marx who convinced many persons that individuals and societies were under the control not of themselves but of the forces of economic order. Sigmund Freud further reduced the area in which contemporary people felt themselves to have authority by developing influential theories regarding the ways in which individuals are at the mercy of psychological forces working within them. The reason for mentioning these thinkers and their challenge to humanity's idea of itself is simply that no patient or nurse is immune to the radical rethinking of humanity's nature and place within the natural order. The very definitions of nature, of health, and, consequently, of illness are directly affected by the work of the major thinkers in fields far outside the conventional limits of health care, such as astronomy, biology, economics and political theory, and psychology and psychoanalysis.

Nurses today have their tasks cut out for them. They have significant moral choices demanded of them. They have to choose whether to "fit in" with models of nursing already developed or take a fresh new look at their field with the intention of making certain it fulfills its high calling as a humane profession the center of which is compassionate, caring advocacy for the patient. They have to choose which image of themselves and their profession they will accept, and to which they will dedicate their professional energies. They cannot pretend such choices do not exist. These choices confront each student of nursing, each practicing nurse, and each nursing educator. Upon the choices the nurses make depend not only their personal careers but also the health of their profession, the health of the health care field itself, and, ultimately, the quality of the health care available to themselves and to all of us.

Endnotes

1. Jo Ann Ashley, *Hospitals, Paternalism and the Role of the Nurse.* (New York: Teachers College Press, 1976), p. 33.

2. *Ibid.*
3. Carol Soares, "Nursing and Medical Diagnoses: A Comparison of Variant and Essential Features," *The Nursing Profession,* ed. Norma L. Chaska (New York: McGraw-Hill, 1978), pp. 269–278.
4. American Council of Learned Societies Statement, cited in W. T. Jones, "What's the Use of the Humanities? A Primer for the Perplexed," *Engineering and Science,* January-February 1977, p. 4.
5. Jones, "What's the Use of the Humanities?" p. 6.
6. Sally Gadow, "Humanistic Issues at the Interface of Nursing and the Community," *Humanistic Studies in Medicine,* June 1977, pp. 357–361.
7. André Malraux, *The Walnut Trees of Altenberg,* cited by Maurice Friedman in *To Deny Our Nothingness* (New York: Delacorte Press, 1967), p. 17.

Should nurses be content to practice today in the familiar paternalistic context? Should they be advocates of patients' rights? Should they see themselves primarily as healers, champions of the poor who are ill, substitute doctors, parents, or counselors? Carrying further the discussion of the previous essays with their concern for developing models of the nurse–patient relation and for establishing a philosophy of the profession, Sally Gadow here develops a philosophy which she calls "existential advocacy." She presents a thoroughly reasoned argument for the rejection of paternalism and of nursing as primarily a matter of championing the rights of patients. Instead, she argues that nursing is concerned—or ought to be—with the whole person of the patient. Obviously, this model of nursing has implications for both the education and the practice of nurses at every level.

3

Existential Advocacy: Philosophical Foundation of Nursing

Sally Gadow

1. Introduction: Against Meta-Nursing

Turning points occur in the history of a profession, when radical questioning and clarification are essential for further growth. We recognize such a turning point now in nursing. The direction in which the basic concept of nursing develops will determine whether the profession draws closer to the model of medicine with its commitment to science, technology and cure, reverts to historical nursing models with their essentially intuitive approaches, or creates a new philosophy which sets contemporary nursing distinctively apart from both traditional nursing and modern medicine.

The question of whether such a distinctive concept of nursing is possible is itself not even resolved, however. One sociologist suggests that, rather than the evolution of a new philosophy of nursing, nurses will evolve out of nursing: "nursing will still be nursing, but it will be carried on by persons of other occupational affiliations."[1] What will nurses be doing while someone else is doing the nursing? They will be moving on to meta-nursing. In the words of one of them, "The role of the nurse must be transcended in order to relate as human being to human being."[2]

Copyright © Stuart F. Spicker, Ph.D. This essay originally appeared in *Nursing: Images and Ideals (Opening Dialogue with the Humanities),* Stuart F. Spicker and Sally Gadow (Eds.), Springer Publishing Co., 1980, pp. 79–101. We are grateful to Stuart Spicker and the Springer Publishing Co. for permission to reprint the article in its entirety.

If nursing is conceptualized in such a way that it must be transcended in order to involve the nurse as a human being, it is not surprising that nurses relinquish some of their functions to other health workers. The fact, however, that they nevertheless consider themselves nurses suggests that the meta-nursing to which they turn is *not* a transcending or outgrowing of nursing but an early expression, not yet explicit, of new possibilities within nursing.

This simple phenomenon, that persons who have, in the sociologist's eyes, moved beyond nursing still consider themselves nurses, reflects the belief which is the premise of this paper: that nursing is to be defined philosophically rather than sociologically, defined by the (ideal) nature and purpose of the nurse-patient relation rather than by a specific set of behaviors. When the concept of nursing is addressed as a philosophical ideal rather than an empirical construct, we see immediately that it is contradictory to speak of nurses transcending nursing or delegating it to non-nurses. If nursing, in other words, is distinguished by its philosophy of care and not by its care functions, and if nurses themselves formulate that philosophy, they transcend a particular concept of nursing only in order to realize a more developed concept, an ideal: a philosophy of nursing which unifies and enhances the experience of the individuals involved rather than devaluing and alienating any of that experience.

The candidates for an ideal concept of nursing are familiar to anyone acquainted with the history of nursing: the nurse as healer, champion of the sick poor, parent-surrogate, physician-surrogate, contracted clinician, personal counselor, and health educator, among others. The concept which I will propose as the philosophical foundation and ideal of nursing is that of advocacy—not the concept of advocacy implied in the patient's rights movement, in which any health professional is potentially a consumer advocate, but a fundamental, existential advocacy for which the nurse alone, among all of the health professionals, is uniquely suited, and which is as distinct from consumerism as it is from paternalism.

The concept of existential advocacy proposed here is not simply one more alternative in the list of past and present concepts of nursing, nor does it imply a rejection of all other concepts. Rather, it is proposed as the philosophical foundation upon which the patient and nurse in any given encounter can freely decide whether their relation shall be that of child-and-patient, client-and-counselor, friend-and-friend, colleague-and-colleague, and so on through the range of possibilities. Thus, the foundation of existential advocacy is philosophically prior to (i.e., the ground of the possibility for) freely determining, within an actual nurse–patient relation, the form that relation is to have.

In elaborating the proposed ideal of advocacy, I will first distinguish the concept from both paternalism and patient's rights advocacy. I will then describe advocacy nursing as a philosophical as well as concrete resolution of two related conflicts within health care which manifest in nursing the greatest urgency and the greatest possibility for solution: the dichotomy between the personal and the professional within the health care provider, and the discrepancy between the lived body and the object body within the patient. Finally, I will propose that existential advocacy, as the essence of nursing, is the nurse's participation with the patient in determining the unique meaning which the experience of health, illness, suffering or dying is to have for that individual.

2. Conceptual Framework

The meaning of advocacy nursing which I will develop in this paper must be distinguished from paternalism and consumerism, both of which are sometimes confused with a notion of patient advocacy.

The conflict in health care between advocacy and paternalism is felt most acutely by the nurse, who must reconcile nursing's traditional alliance with the patient and its modern allegiance to medicine. Moreover, humanistic and author-itarian tendencies compete in nursing with particular intensity because of the comprehensive yet personal nature of the care given. The nurse attends the individual as a unity rather than a single problem or system; attends the in-dividual when distress is immediate and the patient the most vulnerable; and attends the individual during periods of sustained contact, often providing the mundane intimacies usually considered to be self-care. Thus the nurse is in the ideal position among health care providers to experience the patient as a unique human being with individual strengths and complexity—a precondition for advocacy. On the other hand, the potential for paternalism is as great as that for advocacy, for just those reasons. The comprehensiveness, immediacy and continuity of care present an exceptional opportunity for powerful influence over individuals—the precondition for paternalism.

a. Paternalism

The concept of advocacy proposed here is in essence the opposite of paternalism. For that reason, it is important to clearly formulate the meaning of paternalism which is being used.

Paternalistic acts (and attitudes) are those which limit the liberty or rights of individuals in their own interests. Implied in the notion of restricting another's freedom, or infringing upon rights, is the element of coercion (since individuals who voluntarily submit to a restriction are theoretically exercising their liberty in that choice). A more explicit meaning of paternalism, then, is the use of coercion to provide a good that is not desired by the one whom it is intended to benefit.[3]

It has been argued that the essential element in paternalism (other than its motivation, the intent to obtain a good for the person affected) is not coercion, but more broadly "the violation of moral rules, for example, the moral rules prohibiting deception, deprivation of freedom or opportunity, or disabling."[4] But this view fails to account for the case, for example, in which a woman anticipating discovery of a malignancy asks that she not be told if her fears are confirmed, and the physician complies by lying to her. Here a moral rule has been violated in the interest of the person affected, but it is doubtful whether the authors of this view would judge the action paternalistic. On the contrary, overriding the patient's wishes and forcing the truth upon her (if done for her own good) would count as paternalistic.[5] The single moral "rule," then, which is negated by paternalism is the prohibition against coercion, here defined as the forcing of individuals either to act in some way that is contrary to their wishes or to submit to an action of another that is contrary to their wishes. (An example of the former is the requirement that even unwilling students write examinations; of the latter, the insistence that uncooperative patients submit to any diagnostic procedures the practitioner believes necessary.)

In summary, there are two principal elements in paternalism: (1) the intent: obtaining what is believed to be a good for the other person; (2) the effect: violating the person's known wishes in the matter.

The meaning of paternalism is formulated differently by its defenders, not in terms of violation but assistance. That view expresses the belief that in matters affecting an individual's well-being, for the person's own good decisions should be made by those most capable of knowing what actions are in the person's interest.[6] Accordingly, it is inherent in professional responsibility always to act in the patient's interest. Paternalism is not a violation of the patient's right of self-determination as much as it is a protection of the patient's right to the best possible care that can be given.

This positive interpretation of paternalism only confuses matters, however, by reducing paternalism to an identity with an equally simplistic meaning of advocacy, viz. acting on behalf of another. With this confusion, the most paternalistic professional can claim to be the staunchest patient advocate. (Indeed, paternalism becomes the most thoroughgoing form of advocacy, inasmuch as it goes the length of even opposing individuals' wishes in order to act in their interest.) The conflation of paternalism and advocacy is a confusion which negates the truth of both, viz. that paternalism is a violation of the right of self-determination, and that advocacy does not consist in acting on another's behalf. The two are philosophically contradictory concepts.

b. Consumerism

If advocacy and paternalism are opposites, does this mean that advocacy reduces to the professional's doing whatever the patient wishes (since paternalism amounts to the patient's doing whatever the professional wishes)? Is advocacy a form of consumer protection, in which the role of the professional is to provide information necessary for the patient's informed selection among available courses of action? Is the advocate nurse a technical advisor whose responsibility stops short of recommending one option over another, lest that recommendation become coercion?

The answer to these is no, for professional consumerism is but a sophisticated form of paternalism, which insists that, in the interest of individuals' autonomy, they be forced to make important decisions with only technical assistance, i.e., information about their options. The fact that information is provided which has traditionally been denied to patients does not alter the paternalistic assumption that that is all that should be provided in order for patients to act autonomously—nor, for that matter, the assumption that individuals ought to act autonomously.

The current concept of patients' rights advocacy should be understood in this light, as a species of the wider movement of consumerism. "Patient advocacy is seeing that the patient knows what to expect and what is his right to have, and then displaying the willingness and courage to see that our system does not prevent his getting it."[7] On this view, the advocate is, at worst, the equivalent of a "bill of rights" brochure in the patient's hands; at best, a troubleshooter willing to intervene when the system violates an individual's rights.[8]

c. Advocacy

The concept of existential advocacy (which will be intended from this point on whenever the term "advocacy" is used) is distinct from both paternalism and consumer protection. It is based upon the principle that freedom of self-determination is the most fundamental and valuable human right, and therefore is a greater good than any which health care can provide.

In negative terms, this implies that the right of self-determination ought not be infringed even in the interest of health. The professional, while obligated to act in the patient's interest, is not permitted to define that interest in any way contrary to the patient's definition: it is not the professional but the patient who determines what "best interest" shall mean.

In positive terms, this meaning of advocacy has far greater implications for the professional, which extend beyond the narrow realm of proscriptions into the realm of ideals. The ideal which existential advocacy expresses is this: that individuals be *assisted* by nursing to *authentically* exercise their freedom of self-determination. By authentic is meant a way of reaching decisions which are truly one's own—decisions that express all that one believes important about oneself and the world, the entire complexity of one's values.

Individuals can express their wholeness and uniqueness as valuing beings only if their full complexity of values—including contradictions and conflicts— is clearly in mind, having been re-examined and clarified in the new context. Yet, that clarification is the most difficult exactly when it is most needed, when a situation arises which threatens to overturn previously stable values. In such situations, of which health impairment is a paradigm, individuals face the necessity of either recreating their values or recreating their situation according to their existing hierarchy of values. The paternalistic response to this is simple: Never mind examining values, because health is the highest human value. The response of consumerism to the patient is still more simple: Once you have been informed of all your options, do whatever you like.

The response of advocacy differs from both of these. It is not based on an assumption about what individuals *should want* to do, nor does it consist in protecting individuals' *right* to do what they want. It is the effort to help persons *become clear about what they want* to do, by helping them discern and clarify their values in the situation, and on the basis of that self-examination, to reach decisions which express their reaffirmed, perhaps recreated, complex of values. Only in this way, when the valuing self is engaged and expressed in its entirety, can a person's decision be actually *self*-determined instead of being a decision which merely is not determined by others. [9]

3. Advocacy and Contradictions in the Nurse–Patient Relation

Two central contradictions in health care prevent authentic self-determination, despite the lip-service paid to "patient autonomy". They are the dichotomies between personal and professional involvement of the practitioner, and between the lived body and the object body of the patient. Because both of these conflicts result in fragmentation of patient as well as the practitioner, their effect is to seriously limit the extent of the person that is involved in making decisions. If nursing is to accomplish its purpose in existential advocacy—i.e., if patients are to be assisted in making decisions which are genuinely their own because they fully express their own reaffirmed or recreated values—then nursing must resolve both of these contradictions. As long as either remains, a source of self-alienation and personal disunity, the patient is effectively prevented from exercising his or her right of self-determination.

a. *Personal versus Professional*

The movement of humanistic health care has attempted to soften the contradiction between the person and the professional. Professionals are encouraged to become involved with and attentive to patients as individuals—in other words, to behave more like persons than professionals—while patients have begun to assume some of the responsibilities formerly reserved for the professional.

But the dichotomy persists, nevertheless. In all health professions, young practitioners are warned that becoming personally involved with patients is unprofessional (in spite of patients' complaints that their care is too impersonal). The traditional view maintains that the personal and the professional are mutually exclusive aspects of the practitioner: behaving professionally entails avoidance of any personal interactions, i.e., behavior expressing the professional's feelings, values, or idiosyncracies. On this view, individuals are interchangeable, because none of their individuality is allowed into their interactions with patients.

Another version of this view considers the professional role to be one among many in which the person engages. Different elements of the person are distributed among the various roles, with the result that at least something of the individual is expressed in professional behavior. That "something", however, usually includes at most the person's scientific, technical, and managerial capabilities; the emotional, aesthetic, and contemplative, among others, are confined to other domains of the person's life.

Both of these views have the inevitable effect of fragmenting the individual, the nurse, who guards against any 'leaking' of the personal domains into the professional. Because of that exclusion of significant elements of the person from the professional relation, self-estrangement occurs within the nurse and, consequently, within the patient. Regarding the patient as a "whole" requires nothing less than the nurse acting as a "whole" person; therefore, the nurse who withholds parts of the self is unlikely to allow the patient to emerge as a whole (or to comprehend that wholeness if it does emerge).

Are we justified in assuming that the traditional view is right, that one essential feature of 'professional' is its exclusion of the personal? In different terms, does the introduction of the personal into the professional domain so alter the nature of 'professional' that its distinctiveness disappears and it becomes essentially no different than giving help to a friend or to oneself?

To answer, we can examine phenomenologically the differences between patient and professional in a hypothetical situation—the relation between, for example, two women who are professional colleagues, one of whom provides nursing care for the other. In such a relation between professional equals, any non-essential differences (such as expertise) disappear, and it should be possible to discern only essential differences. (To further avoid confusion with non-essential differences, we can stipulate that the colleague designated as the care provider suffers from the same disease as the person receiving care.) Here, the two persons relating to one another as patient and nurse have a comparable understanding of the health problem in question; there is no difference in their competence to deal with the disease as a clinical entity. The essential differences arise with respect to their dealing with the illness as a personal experience. Those differences can be classified in terms of (1) focus, (2) intensity, and (3) perspective.

(1) The focus of the patient is directed to the problem at hand and its effect upon her life; her concern is unavoidably self-oriented. The focus of the professional, in contrast, is directed away from herself toward the other. Her feelings of distress over the other's pain may be expressed, but not in order to obtain relief thereby or receive help from the patient. There is not, as in personal relations, a mutuality in which both are equally concerned about the other, with each one also maintaining some degree of self-interest. In the professional relation, the practitioner is interested in the other's good more than her own, while the patient is concerned primarily about her well-being rather than the other's.

Personal relations too, though fundamentally relations of mutuality, can assume a one-directional focus when one of the persons is in distress, but two important differences remain between that situation and the professional relation. In friendship, mutuality is the accepted ideal, and departures from it when one or the other person needs unusual attention are understood to be temporary, whereas the basis of the professional relation is the permanent disposition of one of the persons to attend to the other without receiving attention in return. Furthermore, in personal relations, because of the ideal of mutuality, there is a point beyond which a onesided focus becomes unacceptable, and the relation must either return to a reciprocal one or dissolve. In the professional relation, such a limit does not exist, inasmuch as the professional does not depend upon receiving the attention of the patient to make the relationship worthwhile.

(2) The intensity of the situation is experienced differently by the professional and the patient. The latter is caught up in the immediacy of her distress, the urgency of the symptoms as compelling phenomena in themselves. The professional may feel the same urgency (particularly when she has experienced the symptoms herself), but she is not bound by their immediacy. Her continued focus upon the other entails that she remain at the level of reflection rather than feeling, in order to integrate feelings and knowledge in attempting to alleviate the other's distress and thereby free the patient from her confinement to the immediate. Thus it is the form and direction, not the degree, of intensity which necessarily differ in the two persons.

This difference in intensity can occur in personal relations as well, but, like the onesided focus described in (1), it is a departure from the ideal of mutuality, in which the intensity of one's experience is fully shared in its immediacy by the other before becoming the object of reflection. In the professional relation, the intensity felt by the nurse is not a sharing with the patient which has value in itself, value that is independent of helping the other; rather, the intensity serves as an intensification of the reflective process necessary for help to be given. Being able to help has greater value than simply sharing the other's experience—an inversion of the values in personal relations.

(3) In addition to differences in focus and intensity, the perspectives of the two persons differ. The professional is "externally" involved, despite the similarities between herself and the patient, whereas the patient is involved in a radically interior way, feeling the pain "from the inside" and knowing that, although others may have the same disease, it is only *her* body which is affected in this instance.

This is the difference usually designated as the nurse's objectivity and the patient's subjectivity. Unfortunately, these terms are often used specifically to indicate degrees of emotional involvement. The implication is that the essential difference in the two persons' perspectives is that the patient is more, the nurse less, emotional. This ignores the possibility that both persons experience emotional intensity (even though, in the professional, that intensity does not remain at the level of immediacy, but acts as an intensification of other dimensions of the person).

The essential difference in the perspectives of the two persons is related, not to emotion, but to the body. Only the patient can experience her body as an interiority, a living subjectivity, and only someone other than the patient can experience her body as a technical object, a thing to be regarded strictly scientifically.

Because patient and nurse have fundamentally different modes of access to the patient's body, and thus experience it in opposite ways, their understanding of it differs. The patient understands her body as a unique reality that cannot be expressed through types or generalizations. The nurse understands the patient's body as essentially part of the world of objects and therefore most effectively approached through clinical categories. She is of course ultimately concerned with the patient as a unique human being, but she addresses the body's phenomena as instances of general types of phenomena. "Pain here" is categorized as "gastralgia" in order to apply the appropriate remedy. In short, in their involvement with the patient's body, the patient is oriented toward uniqueness, the professional toward typification.

The patient herself, as a professional whose involvement with patients' bodies is characteristically oriented toward the general, can to some extent combine the general with the unique in considering her own body. But because both approaches are required in ideal health care, each one needs to be developed as fully as possible, and this the person alone cannot do, even in her dual role as patient and professional. The two orientations, though complementary, are categorically different, and the patient in most cases engages in one only by diminishing her engagement in the other. For the two perspectives to be thoroughly utilized together, a second person is needed to develop the objective dimension.

Again, the question arises whether the second person need be a professional, or could as well be a friend. Here, as in the differences in focus and intensity, the value of mutuality in personal relations prevents the friend from maintaining a onesided approach, except as a temporary departure from supporting the other as an ultimately indivisible unity of subject and object. The professional, unlike the friend or the patient herself, is able to maintain for the patient the one perspective toward her experience which is the most difficult for her to develop: sustained objectivity.

In considering these three differences between personal and professional relations, and between the patient and the professional, we see that the most commonly assumed difference is absent: the nurse's manifesting less involvement as a whole person than is manifested by patient or friend. On the contrary, the differences described above suggest that, while the form and direction of involvement differ significantly, the 'amount' of the person involved is equally great.

On that basis, a resolution of the personal/professional dichotomy can be proposed in the following way. Professional involvement is not an alternative to other kinds of involvement, such as emotional, aesthetic, physical, or intellectual. It is a deliberate synthesis of all of these, a participation of the *entire* self, using every dimension of the person as a resource in the professional relation.

The concept of professional involvement as a unifying and directing of one's *entire* self in relation to another's need is entailed by the concept of existential advocacy. That concept implies that patients can be assisted in reaching decisions which express their complex totality as individuals only by nurses who themselves act out of the same explicit self-unity, allowing no dimension of themselves to be exempt from the professional relation. Furthermore, the nurse, among health professionals, is uniquely able to actualize such a holistic view of the professional. Nursing care, because of its immediate, sustained, and often intimate nature, as well as its scientific and ethical complexity, offers ready avenues for every dimension of the professional to be engaged, including the emotional, rational, aesthetic, intuitive, physical, and philosophical.

One objection is commonly raised against resolving the personal/professional dichotomy in this way. It is that the professional's emotional involvement (for example) entails for the patient the risk of biased clinical judgment and for the professional the risk of personal suffering and emotional depletion. Such an objection, however, is based on a seriously limited view of emotional involvement. It assumes that through the feeling of another's suffering, "suffering itself becomes infectious."[10] In other words, to participate in another's emotion and have direct knowledge of it is to experience that emotion oneself and be as bound by its immediacy as the person originally experiencing it.

A significantly different possibility for emotional involvement which that view does not consider is the experience of "fellow-feeling" described by Max Scheler. Fellow-feeling is distinct from emotional infection and from merely perceiving the other's emotion. "It is indeed a case of *feeling* the other's feeling, not just knowing it, nor judging that the other has it; but it is not the same as going through the experience itself."[11]

The distinction between fellow-feeling and emotional infection, or identification, reflects the same difference described earlier in relation to the different focus and intensity of patient and professional. The focus of fellow-feeling is the *other's* feeling, not one's own, which prevents emotional participation from becoming infectious identification. The emotion of the patient is not merely reproduced or re-enacted within the professional (making the latter the one needing help). Rather, the patient's feeling is "vicariously visualized" in order to make possible a *"directing* of feeling towards the other's joy or suffering."[12] To participate in the suffering of the other in fact precludes my producing suffering in myself, since then my own experience—not the patient's—would be the object of my focus.

The difference of intensity is related to that difference of focus. In fellow-feeling in contrast to emotional identification (i.e., in the professional's feeling as distinct from the patient's), the intensity is consciously directed, whereas in the experiencing of one's own emotion or the identification with another's, involvement is immediate rather than directed, involuntary rather than deliberate, and often unconscious. It is the failure to distinguish this different intensity of fellow-feeling from emotional identification which gives rise to the objection that emotional involvement distorts professional judgment. In emotional infection the nurse indeed succumbs to the same involuntary and unconscious immediacy which the patient experiences, and it could be argued that that use of intensity might well distort judgment. But fellow-feeling is a different, *directed* intensity, "a genuine *out-reaching* and entry into the other person and his individual situation, a true and authentic transcendence of one's self."[13]

Fellow-feeling is but one example of the concrete resolution possible in advocacy nursing: resolution of the personal/professional dichotomy, in this case by the nurse's deliberate emotional participation with the patient. For the patient's emotional complexity to be understood and supported, the emotional dimension of the nurse's own being cannot be excluded, but must be consciously, directly engaged. Moreover, just as with the emotional, so too the aesthetic, intuitive, physical, philosophical, and all other dimensions of personal reality can and must be brought to bear as essential, positive elements in the professional relation.[14] The absolute prerequisite for advocacy—advocating the patient's own individually created values—is the participation of the advocate as an individual, a complete unity unfragmented by exclusion of any part of the self.

b. Lived Body versus Object Body

The traditional dichotomy in the experience of the nurse between personal and professional involvement is directly related to the dichotomy in the experience of the patient between the body as a private, lived reality and a public object open to inspection. The nurse's personal involvement with patients has been assumed to interfere with professional functions. Similarly, the patient's orientation toward the subjective body has been assumed to contradict the clinical orientation toward the body as an object. Thus the concept of the professional as impersonal and objective has dictated a corresponding way of regarding the patient's body, viz. as object rather than person.

A paradigm of the sharp contradiction within the patient's experience of her body is the gynecological examination, in which a strictly impersonal definition is in force. For the patient, the part of the body being examined is often an extremely personal part of the self, perhaps the most private and emotionally invested part of the body. In the clinical situation, "the pelvic area is like any other part of the body," i.e., the individual examining the patient is "working on a technical object and not a person."[15] Any deviation from the technical attitude, e.g., by a patient's embarassment, is countered with a repertoire of professional nonchalance, concentration on the procedure itself, and assurances that the situation is quite routine (and thus non-intimate).

In the gynecological examination, the patient experiences an abrupt contradiction between her body as her own individual reality, rich with private emotional associations, and her body as sheer object, which others examine as impersonally as a technician examines a machine. That contradiction, in less dramatic form, is fundamental throughout health care, and because it can be uniquely resolved in nursing, it is important to analyze its elements and development here.

The distinction between lived and object body was indirectly indicated earlier in the discussion of the opposite perspectives of patient and professional toward the body of the patient. The distinction there was described in terms of uniqueness versus typification. That formulation expresses one aspect of the opposition, which can now be elaborated more fully.

The object body is the simpler of the two concepts for health professionals to appreciate. It is the body which the anatomist and physiologist describe, an object fully accessible upon examination and fully comprehensible by its examiner. It belongs, as do all objects, to the dimensions of quantified space and time, and to the realm of the general, the category. It is an object whose parts have only functional value, and not emotional, aesthetic, or spiritual value: in the object body the stomach has greater value than the hands of the concert pianist, the eyes of the painter, the legs of the dancer.

The lived body is existentially opposed to the object body, but *is not its opposite*. The lived body is not the silence of the object body when functioning well, so that I am unconscious of its objective existence as long as nothing in it breaks down (in the same way that I am unconcerned with my car's operation as long as no startling noises break into my consciousness). That unawareness of the body is not the lived body; it is simply a negative contingency, an experience conditional upon my not encountering the body-as-object. As a positive condition categorically independent of and experientially prior to consciousness of the body-as-object, the lived body is not a thing at all (not even a well-running, non-intrusive thing), such as we usually denote by the word "body". Thus it cannot be the opposite of the object body. It is instead a mode of orientation: the immediate, prereflective consciousness of the self *as capable of affecting its world,* as well as the consciousness of being vulnerable.[16]

With this understanding of the lived body as independent of and prior to the experience of the object body, it is not only not necessary, it is not allowable, to employ the concept of physical to describe the way in which the self acts and the world in which it acts. It is equally inappropriate to describe the lived body as uniquely mine, for this too places it on the level of the object body. There is meaning in speaking of the object body as mine, because that can be distinguished from its being not-mine, and there is a sense in which my body as object is not fully mine, does not express my purposes, even prevents my acting. But the lived body cannot be "mine", for there is no sense in which it can ever be not-mine; it is *I myself,* a way of being-in-the-world, not a piece of the physical world which (at times) belongs to me.

If the lived body is not a material entity, it is also not in objective space and time. On the contrary, it forms its own space through its actions, drawing the world's space toward it, so to speak, centripetally.[17] Nearness and distance are a function of relevance, not measure. In the same way the lived body shapes its own time, with retension and protension interwoven and overlapping according to one's purposes, unconstrained by linearity.

It might be supposed that the lived body could be described (at least metaphorically) as an experience of interiority, but this fails for two reasons. In the first place, empirically, when the distinction between inner and outer emerges—in early childhood and in illness, for example,—it is often the interior of the body which is felt to be 'other', a baffling region not recognized as part of the self in the way that familiar external features and functions are.[18] Secondly, and more important, the lived body is the self in which inner and outer *are not distinguished:* "Being-for-itself must be wholly body and it must be wholly consciousness; it can not be *united* with a body."[19] The metaphor of interiority connotes subjectivity, privacy, privileged access—features implying hiddenness and assuming another, external, part of the self which is exposed. The lived body is thus reduced to a version (inversion) of the object body, its mirror image, when in fact it is another order of being than the object body.

If we understand the concepts of lived and object body as existentially opposed but not as logical opposites, then it is possible to recognize that the destruction of one does not automatically invoke the other (as in "if not a, then b"). It is especially important for the purposes of this paper to recognize the transition that occurs. The immediacy of the lived body is only partly mediated by illness, injury, pain. With the appearance of incapacity, I experience the body as something which opposes my purposes, a weighted mass, a thing-like other which defies and dismays me. Incapacity shatters the lived body. But the transition is not yet complete. The object body does not replace the lived body through illness alone. The otherness of the body in illness is rendered complete only through the category—the most essential instrument of medical science. The clinical category transforms my "pain here" into precise pathological phenomena which—even if I myself am a clinician—have for me no experiential relation to "pain here". The clinical view presents me with a body that is not mine, a disease process of which I have no direct perception. But, though it escapes *my* consciousness, the new reality is "objectively discernible for *others*. Others have informed me of it, others can diagnose it; it is present for others even though I am not conscious of it."[20]

This then is the contradiction generated for the patient, first by the experience of incapacity and, second, by the perspective of science. What unique possibility exists in nursing for reconciling the opposition and restoring to the patient the unity of self which is prerequisite for true self-determination?

The history of professionalism in nursing suggests that nursing has focused exclusively upon the lived body and the object body in turn, moving from the earlier concern for the immediate comfort of the patient, to the modern concern of science for the objective condition of the patient. Nursing can now surpass both of these extremes: the nurse, as advocate of the patient's wholeness, is committed to advocacy of neither the shattered lived body nor the duly imposed object body. Nursing can, in short, make possible for the patient an enrichment of the lived body by the object body, and an enlivening of the object body by the lived body. The nurse can assist the patient to recover the objectified body at a new level at which it is neither mute immediacy nor pure otherness, but an otherness-made-mine, a lived objectness.

The experience of incapacity brings an awareness of the body as a being in its own right, with an irreducible reality of its own, an integrity and givenness that, so to speak, will not be compromised. Denial of that essential fact of human existence is bought at great price: the lost possibility for enriching the self through integration of that otherness.

It is this integration, a conscious unifying of self and body, which advocacy nursing assists the individual to achieve. The nurse assists me, the patient, to live my objectness as my own, instead of allowing it to remain alien. That unity which I achieve is more fully expressive of my totality than even the lived body was. The new unity is a reflective, more complex and articulated reality, inasmuch as I am now able to establish a conscious identification with aspects of my being which were previously undifferentiated, but have, through illness and objectivity, made themselves known. It is now important and possible to make them mine, to an extent that was not important at the level of the object body and was not possible at the level of the lived body. "What threatens to estrange itself in us communicates to us *all the more. . .* that it is actually our own."[21]

It is that reconciliation of the person with the body-as-other, at a new level of integration and articulation, which nursing advocates. Nursing is uniquely able to mediate the lived/object body duality, inasmuch as it addresses both aspects of the person as one. It affirms the value of the lived body through the intimacy of physical care and comforting. At the same time it affirms the reality of the object body by interpreting to patients their experience in terms of an objective framework (usually science, in Western cultures) which enables them to relate an otherwise hopelessly unique and solitary experience to a wider, general understanding. By continuously interrelating the two dimensions, the nurse demonstrates for the patient that the lived/object body relation is not an either/or but a dialectic in which neither aspect is meaningful without the other. Both are essential, and mutually reciprocal.

This is easiest to realize when persons adhere exclusively to one or the other extreme. The modern example is the patient whose entire reality is the object body, who regards and refers to the body only in clinical terms—X-ray findings, laboratory studies, biopsy report, etc. The more common example (given the traditional refusal to allow patients such access to their object bodies) is the patient whose only reality is the lived body, who categorically renounces the object body as alien to the self by designating the health professional the executor for this unwanted estate.

The challenge to advocacy nursing is to enable the individual to reclaim the aspect that has been excluded. Without incorporation of the object body, the lived body is an existentially weightless "I", unmediated and unenriched by detail, function, form. Without the "I" of the lived body, the object body is an inanimate machine belonging to no one and everyone. The ideal of nursing is thus to enable patients to achieve a reconciliation, a re-integration, of these equally one-sided dimensions, in a synthesis that will necessarily be unique for each individual, and without which the self-unity required for patients' authentic self-determination will be impossible.

4. Advocacy and the Right to Meaning

The preceding sections have described existential advocacy in three ways, as:

- the nurse's assistance to individuals in exercising their right of self-determination, through decisions which express the full and unique complexity of their values;
- a mode of involvement with persons which necessarily engages the entire self of the nurse;
- assistance to patients in unifying the experience of the lived body and the object body at a level that incorporates and transcends both.

In conclusion, we can summarize advocacy nursing as the participation with the patient in determining the *personal meaning* which the experience of illness, suffering, or dying is to have for that individual. At no time is the existential concern about the meaning of one's life more urgent than when the nature of continuation of one's existence is in jeopardy. At that point, the crucial question which the individual must answer is not "how can I secure my existence?" but "what does this jeopardy mean?" Only from the answer to that question can decisions then be reached concerning modes of treatment, forms of coping, the degree of autonomy desired, etc. Ultimately, self-determination means the individual's own decision about the meaning which an experience contains, before decisions are reached about responding practically to the experience. For that meaning to be freely determined, it cannot of course be imposed— by the "nature" of the person's condition, by clinical concepts of illness, by professional notions of "loss", "disability", "suffering". Thus, for example, the patient with terminal prostatic carcinoma is free to decide whether he shall think of his experience in moralistic terms (punishment for promiscuity), scientific terms (simple cellular phenomena), cultural terms (permission to grieve), naturalist terms (the inevitable pain and dying that come to all), or purely individual terms which violate all of these—perhaps an inconsolable despair over the absurdity of the experience, or a decision that suffering can be a means of finding one's own way, by confronting the absurdities of existence not as defects but as necessary antitheses in the dialectical relation between joy and sorrow in human life.

For the same reason that the question of meaning arises, viz. the threat to existence, individuals require assistance in determining the meaning that will inform their experience. That assistance is provided ideally by the person who has the most comprehensive understanding of the experience and is as fully involved as the patient. That person is the nurse. The approach of nursing encompasses both care and cure, intimate concern for the lived body and scientific treatment of the object body. Moreover, the nurse offers a necessary alternative perspective which complements and completes the partial perspective of the patient, inasmuch as the focus and intensity of the nurse is directed toward the other rather than the self, and the orientation of the nurse is toward the general rather than the solitary. Finally, the constancy with which only nursing attends the patient enables the nurse to experience individuals as unique human beings continuously engaged in creating their own histories.

No other health profession combines all of these elements. More important, none other even proposes as its *ideal* this reconciliation of the most radical dichotomies in health care: the unique and the general, personal intensity and professional objectivity, the body as "I" and the body as other. Nursing, by aiming at the resolution of these contradictions and the human fragmentation they produce, in order that patient and nurse can participate as unified selves in the patient's process of self-determination, expresses the ideal of existential advocacy. On this basis, the nurse is the ideal professional to participate with the patient in the decision about that which is most crucial in all experiences of illness: the meaning of the experience for the individual.

Endnotes

1. Sam Schulman, "Basic Functional Roles in Nursing: Mother Surrogate and Healer," in *Patients, Physicians, and Illness,* ed. E. Jaco (Glencoe, Illinois: The Free Press, 1958), p. 537, (528-537).
2. Joyce Travelbee, *Interpersonal Aspects of Nursing* (Philadelphia: F. A. Davis, Co., 1966), p. 49.
3. Such a formulation deliberately leaves open whether the person refuses the "good" because it is not recognized as a good, or because its value is lower than other goods in the person's hierarchy of values. The refusal of blood transfusions by Jehovah's Witness patients may reflect, not failure to judge health or life to be a good, but the judging of another end to have a higher value. In either case, interference in that decision is paternalistic. For elaboration of this position, see Dworkin's discussion of Mill in Gerald Dworkin, "Paternalism," *The Monist* 56 (January 1972), pp. 64-84.

4. Bernard Gert and Charles M. Culver, "Paternalistic Behavior," *Philosophy and Public Affairs* 6, no. 1 (Fall 1976), p. 48 (45–57).

5. This in fact is exactly what Gert and Culver argue in regard to a physician's insisting that a patient talk about an impending trauma against her expressed wishes. (*Ibid.*, p. 49).

6. Paternalism thus attributes to the person affected a form of ethical egoism, i.e., the belief that individuals (patients, in this case) *ought* to act in such a way as to promote their own good, with the altruistic footnote that if they fail to do so, action will be initiated on their behalf to obtain the good for them until such time as they resume the moral duties of egoism.

7. Sandra Kosik, "Patient Advocacy or Fighting the System," *American Journal of Nursing*, April 1972, p. 694 (694–698).

8. The goals of patient advocacy programs may not even be solely those of consumer protection. Improving patient compliance and smoothing over patient complaints are often hidden or explicit objectives. Even when the primary goal is helping patients, advocacy can function as a defense for professional decisions: "patients experiencing a token economy wanted to know whether the therapy team was violating patients' rights. . . All it took here was an explanation that token economy is a medically approved, widely accepted, mode of treatment. The patients were more accepting of it after that." (Wanda Nations, "Nurse-Lawyer is Patient-Advocate," *American Journal of Nursing*, June 1973, p. 1039 (1039–1041).

9. Professor Engelhardt's concern here that "paternalism in the interests of health" is being replaced by a "paternalism in the interests of authenticity" is, fortunately, unfounded. I am proposing advocacy as an ideal, not as a duty, norm, prescription, or imperative which conceivably might involve "enforcement." Moreover, it is simply contradictory to believe that we can force persons to act in an unforced way. The ideal of assisting patients to exercise their freedom does not entail that they be stigmatized for declining, just as the ideal of health presumably does not entail that patients be punished for disdaining modern medicine. Authenticity, like health, is ultimately fashioned and confirmed only by the individuals themselves; professionals can assist the process but they cannot command it.

10. Friedrick Nietzsche, *The Anti-Christ*, trans. R. J. Hollingdale (Baltimore: Penguin Books, 1969), p. 118. See also Nietzsche, "The Will to Suffer and Those Who Feel Pity," *The Gay Science*, trans. Walter Kaufman (New York: Random House, 1974), pp. 269–271.

11. Max Scheler, *The Nature of Sympathy*, trans. Peter Heath (Hamdon, Conn.: Archon Books, 1970), p. 9 (emphasis added).

12. *Ibid.*, 15.

13. *Ibid.*, 46.

14. Another example of resolving the personal/professional dichotomy, this time through physical involvement between nurse and patient, can be developed around the importance of touch in nursing. For a discussion of the laying-on of hands in nursing care, see Dolores Krieger, "Therapeutic Touch: The Imprimatur of Nursing," *American Journal of Nursing*, May 1975, pp. 784–787.

15. Joan P. Emerson, "Behavior in Private Place: Sustaining Definitions of Reality in Gynecological Examinations" in *Readings on Ethical and Social Issues in Biomedicine,* ed. Richard W. Wertz (Englewood Cliffs, N. J.: Prentice-Hall, Inc., 1973), pp. 221–223.

16. I am grateful to J. Melvin Moody for his insistance upon the vulnerability of the lived body, elaborated in "Helping the Patient Survive: Some Remarks on Prof. Sally Gadow's Paper 'Existential Advocacy: Philosophical Foundation of Nursing' " (unpublished).

17. Sartre captures this phenomenon of lived space in his analysis of "the look," in which the world is experienced, not as fixed in uniform space, but "perpetually flowing" toward me, its center. (See *Being and Nothingness: An Essay in Phenomenological Ontology*, trans. Hazel Barnes (New York: The Citadel Press, 1969), pp. 232ff.)

18. This is contrary to Sartre's account of the distinction, in which the object body emerges as the exterior part of my self which the other perceives, "extended outside in a dimension of flight which escapes me. My body's depth of being is for me this perpetual 'outside' of my most intimate 'inside' " *Ibid.*, (p. 328).

19. *Ibid.*, 281.

20. Herbert Plügge, "Man and His Body" in *The Philosophy of the Body: Rejections of Cartesian Dualism*, ed. Stuart F. Spicker (New York: Quadrangle/The New York Times Book Co., 1970), p. 305 (292–311).

21. Sartre, *Being and Nothingness*, p. 332.

SECTION

II

The Nurse: Accountability and Role Conflicts

The complexity of the nurse's role in health care institutional settings causes a conflict between many loyalties. The nurse is an employee of the institution and, therefore, accountable to hospital administration. Because of her continuous presence in the daily life of the patient, the nurse carries out many medically delegated tasks in the absence of the physician and is, therefore, accountable to the physician. In addition, nurses as professional practitioners are, above all, accountable to the patient. With the bureaucratization of health care institutions and the increasing technology of medical practice, nurses increasingly find themselves torn between meeting the goals of the institution, the goals of medicine, and the goals of quality nursing care.

In an attempt to serve the best interests of the patient, many nurses are taking the position that they are the patient advocates of the health care system.

The chapters within this unit are oriented toward the conflict of loyalties that nurses face in their daily practice. Anne Davis discusses the sociology of ethics in hospitals and the implications for the ethics of patient care. Given the hierarchical structure of the hospital and the nurse's traditional subservient position within it, Davis raises the question whether or not it is too great a risk for nurses to raise ethical issues or question the behavior of those who are in superior positions.

Alasdair MacIntyre's philosophical analysis of the nurse's dilemma deals with conceptual issues involved in deciding to whom the nurse is responsible. He suggests that before we can say to *whom* the nurse is responsible, we must first answer the question for *what* is the nurse responsible? Maintaining that the current care-cure distinction between nursing and medical functions is not productive and may be an ideological disguise for the dysfunction of the current nurse–physician relationship, he suggests a new function for the nurse as emissary between the two cultures of the patient and physician.

Elsie Bandman raises numerous issues related to patient advocacy and nurse-physician conflict in relation to informed consent and refusal of treatment. Answering the question what it means for the nurse to assure patients' rights, she deals with the dilemma of interfering with the physician's prescribed course of treatment and the right of the nurse to inform patients of alternative, unverified scientific treatment.

Davis examines the sociology of hospital organization and the conflicts its structure and role relationships create. She describes the hospital culture which affects ethical decision making in patient care. The working conditions and frustrations of nurses are discussed and the question is raised whether or not it is ethical for nurses as professional practitioners to engage in collective bargaining for increased decision making and improvement in the quality of patient care.

4

Authority–Autonomy, Ethical Decision Making, and Collective Bargaining in Hospitals

Anne J. Davis

Introduction

Numerous major changes in health care delivery have occurred during this century. One such change, the combination of increased scientific and medical knowledge has led, among other things, to specialization in medicine and nursing. The development of the technological ability to implement this increased knowledge allows health sciences to have more control over life and death now than in previous times. The rapidity of development of knowledge and technology makes apparent that what we consider ordinary and extraordinary health care measures at any given time is relative.

Another factor affecting the delivery of health care in this country, and one which has received less attention in the biomedical literature than the knowledge-technology impact, is the shift from home care, where the family provided for the needs of its sick members who occasionally saw the physician either in an office or in the patient's home, to more institutional care. Medical and social practices caused a great many people in the recent past to view the hospital as a place to go to die, and this was often the case.

The shift to institutional care has greatly affected the nature of professional relations both among those who provide care and between the care givers and the patients. Because of knowledge-technology developments, the development of third-party payments, and the focus on medical specialties, patients now usually receive care and/or cure in institutions with hierarchical division of labor, such as hospitals. This hierarchical division of labor determines roles, functions, and lines of communication of those working in hospitals. This paper examines selected factors in the sociology of ethics in hospitals and the impact these factors have on the role and ethics of the hospital nurse. In addition, some questions regarding collective bargaining for nurses are raised.

Authority-Autonomy and the Physician

At the beginning of the twentieth century, physicians constituted 80 percent of all health workers, whereas today they account for about 12 percent of the total health workforce. Most of these physicians are men and entrepreneurs, while most of the non-physician workers are women and employees. These realities determine the dynamics of hospital care and, importantly, they have implications for the ethics of that care. Social and structural changes have, in turn, changed role definitions and role interplay in hospitals. The discussion in this paper is limited to hospitals because most nurses work in these settings, which provide an easily accessible arena for social science research on these variables of social and structural change. In addition, physicians have become increasingly dependent on hospitals and other health care institutions and organizations to carry out their work. These changes threaten the traditional autonomy of physicians in private practice, because patient care is now given by many different specialized individuals. However, the physician in the hospital setting can still claim expertise over any and all activities in the health care arena. In essence, the physician, the dominant professional, stands in a totally different structural relationship to the division of labor in hospitals than the subordinate does. One important question which arises in this context is: What is the generalized hospital culture, including the value system, which affects ethical decision making? A study by Millman explores selected aspects of this question and illuminates the variety of ways that physicians define, perceive, and respond to their own mistakes and those of their colleagues.[1] In examining the methods doctors use to systematically ignore and justify medical errors or to treat them as inconsequential events, this research concludes that these responses are built into the hospital organization and the physician's professional training and outlook. In addition, the lines of authority and responsibility, even in university-affiliated teaching hospitals, are often sufficiently ambiguous to permit a pervasive lack of control in matters that physicians refer to as the exercise of poor judgment.

According to Millman, what happens is a neutralization of mistakes, a process that fits into the ideology of medical work within the context of special loyalties and group affiliations. Whether a physician defines an activity as a mistake, and how she or he responds to it, depends a great deal upon the operation of conflicting interests and rivalries of different groups of doctors within the hospital. The right to intervene in another doctor's activities, the responsibility for cooperating or participating in another doctor's error, becomes determined by the particular configuration of statuses and specialties of the physicians involved. Ritualized institutional ceremonies neutralize mistakes by fitting them into the organization and ideology of medical work. Such a situation led Millman to conclude that no universal standards of right/wrong or good/bad medical practice determine the ideas, rules, and practices regarding mistakes among physicians. Rather, these standards tend to emerge from the practical interests of each hospital department. The hierarchy formed by the different medical specialties and the various levels of prepared physicians, such as interns, residents, and attendings, also plays a major role in maintaining the lack of any universal standards.

Another factor, documented in recent years, is that the very definition of a medical mistake tends to shift according to the social value of the patient as assessed by the physician. One aspect of this shifting value is in negative labels such as "crocks" or "turkeys" since these patients become defined as undeserving of serious medical attention.[2] Along with this medico-social definition of patient worth, the professional self-concept, functional for both physicians and patients, indicates that physicians tend to view themselves as self-sufficient and self-confident. To the degree that these professional personal characteristics become highly valued, admissions of uncertainty or error are not easily accommodated into such a self-concept. Expressed self-doubt becomes unacceptable. A physician's positive self-presentation is greatly functional for patients who need to view the physician as infallible. Such a combination of factors may serve to close the ranks among health care givers and to limit patient autonomy.

The general public tends to believe that physicians are guided almost totally by scientific objectivity, but most medical situations are more complex than that. For example, what by definition constitutes sickness, what constitutes appropriate treatment, how such treatment should be given, what patients should be told, along with which alternatives should be offered do not necessarily arise from neutral scientific evidence alone, but from perspectives and definitions of the situation that reflect, among other things, the individual's interest and position. This does not mean that biases stem from bad intentions, but it does acknowledge that defining the situation depends in very large part on particulars and limited experiences and interests. The physician's perspective and the extent to which this perspective protects his or her own interests rather than always serving those of the patient must be examined. Even with the best of intentions, is it possible that some physicians perceive the hospital as being there to make their work easier and/or more profitable? Physicians do not differ from members of other groups in some basic ways, but because of their unusual privilege and power in our society, the special obligations in their work, and the historical nature of the patient role, doctors' behavior and beliefs are not often questioned or challenged before the fact. After-the-fact malpractice suits reflect not only basic incompetence, in some cases, but also the interplay of the physician's professional self-concept with the often unrealistic expectations patients have of physicians and their abilities and powers.

Other Health Personnel in Hospitals

Specific social and role constraints affecting other hospital personnel are limited to three interrelated factors: (1) sex-linked occupations, (2) formal and informal patterns of influence and power, and (3) employee status. Manpower in today's health field is womanpower since 75 percent of all health workers are women. These groups have so much responsibility for the daily necessities of patient care that they are an important dynamic in the formerly private relationship between patient and physician. Because more hospital personnel either witness or participate in medical events, medical practice has become a more public event. An audience, either immediate or potential, has the potential to change both the dynamics and content of the interaction between physicians and patients and has ramifications for other hospital personnel.

In examining social roles in hospitals the fact that the majority of the personnel are women and employees must be considered. Medicine, as a professional group, dominates the health delivery system, supported by the greater knowledge and accountability of physicians. At the same sime, however, medicine has become increasingly dependent on non-physician groups, referred to by some social scientists as semi-professionals characterized by a lack of strong reference group orientation to colleagues and, therefore, without a generalized colleague group as a source of norms. This situation maintains the status quo of the hierarchy among physicians and other health care personnel because these semi-professional groups are more willing to accept an administrative superior as their norm source. Simpson believes that this pattern is due to the prevalence of women in the semi-professions who can be characterized as more amenable to administrative control, less conscious of organizational status, and more submissive in this context than men.[3]

Women, socialized in our society, have historically been placed in a secondary position. To the extent that this discrimination continues, it affects social situations in hospitals. These so-called semi-professionals such as nurses assist the physician in scientific tasks and function to overcome inadequacies in the medical scientific method. One way they do this is to prevent knowledge of error from reaching the patient and her or his family. Essentially, these semi-professional groups are expected to react with moral passivity to their knowledge of hospital events.[4] If we accept that such expectations exist, we can assume that nurses who continue to work in hospitals are either comfortable with this state of affairs or experience low morale and burn-out. If either is the case, we can further assume that involvement in and concern about one's own and others' ethical or unethical decisions can easily be viewed as beyond the call of duty.

These comments focused on non-physician hospital personnel are not intended to imply that these are evil people interacting with the world in bad faith. Given the organizational structure of hospitals, the division of labor, and the hierarchical ordering of personnel, social constraints are built in to the hospital system.

In hospitals when an individual worker or a group comes to grips with an ethical dilemma, the risk/benefit ratio of the formal and informal reward/punishment system operating in the institution often comes into play. The major question becomes: Can semi-professional employees who function within this social structure as buffers between the bureaucratic system and the patient risk raising ethical issues, especially if these issues involve those in superior positions within the system?

Emile Durkheim makes the point that professionals are part of a moral community. Social links develop not only to their clients and colleagues in their own profession, but also to other groups with whose activities their skills must dovetail. The legitimacy of their contribution, however, must be acknowledged by others.[5] Being labeled "semi-professional" can inhibit such acknowledgment, maintain the formal power structure, and impede vital interchange on ethical and other issues central to good health care.

The American Nurses' Association Code for Nurses

The American Nurses' Association Code for Nurses represents one major means for nursing to exercise professional self-regulation.[6] Its basic stance is that the nurse is accountable to the patient. In saying that "neither physician's prescriptions nor the employing agency's policies relieves the nurse of ethical or legal accountability for actions taken and judgments made," the Code either dismisses or bypasses the fact that most nurses work in situations in which they experience multiple loyalties—to the institution, to the physician, to themselves as nurses, and to themselves as individuals with value systems. In the abstract, one can only agree with the Nurses' Association's stance. In reality, however, one needs to raise some questions. For example, does the nursing profession organized through its association have any responsibility to aid nurses who do take ethical stances and come into conflict with either an institution or a physician? Recently, a nurse employed in a hospital was assigned to a critical care unit but refused this assignment because she said that she had not worked in this setting and was not safe. The hospital fired this nurse for taking an ethical stance on what she considered to be unsafe practice. The hospital's outmoded concept of "coverage by floating" reflects a simpler time when all nurses were generalists and most units of the hospital could function adequately with this type of nurse. This is no longer always the case due to increased knowledge and technology as mentioned earlier. Given the fact that hospitals must cover units for patient care, and given the fact that the code of nursing ethics encourages nurses to be accountable to patients and, as a baseline, provide safe care, what, if any, responsibility does the official nursing association have toward its members who take such a stance? Do the institutions in which nurses practice have an obligation to take seriously the nursing code of ethics? Under the current institutional structural arrangements, can they afford ethical nurses? Can they afford to have such nurse practitioners?

Nursing and the Health Care Industry

In 1972, the employed nursing force in this country contained 780,000 registered nurses, 427,000 practical nurses or LVNs (licensed vocational nurses),
and approximately 900,000 others, such as nursing aides and orderlies. These
numbers of care givers total 2,107,000 people or about 48 percent of the 4.4
million people employed in our health industry. Importantly, this group constitutes about 68 percent of the health workers rendering direct aid to patients.

The financial gains of hospital, nursing home, and other health care facility
employers are derived from the surplus value of labor of these nursing workers.
These employers utilize the services of these wage earners and at the same time
pocket the health care fees paid by the consumers. The high incomes of physicians are, to some extent, due to the medical profession's restriction of its own
labor supply as well as its power and entrepreneur status. But the major source
of the high profits and incomes of the elite generally in the health care industry
lies in the work of the nursing labor force. Without these workers, the employers
in the health care system would be unable to market the mass of health services
from which they make their financial gains and by which they maintain their
power.

The nursing force, because it occupies a key position in the actual delivery of
health care, is in a potentially powerful position to keep health employers from
maintaining that control. In our society, the subjugation of the masses of
workers in the interests of the private gain of those few who control the means
of labor, in essence, can be viewed as the denial of workers' rights to control
the use of their own labor. These rights will probably only come to those workers who collectively develop sufficient political power to take control of their
own work processes.

To put these comments in context, the health care delivery industry has
become big business. The total expenditure in the United States for health and
medical care in 1950 was 12 billion dollars; in 1965, fifteen years later, it had
more than tripled to 38.9 billion dollars. In 1971, the total was 83.4 billion
dollars annually. In short, during a period of twenty-one years, the annual
expenditure for health and medical care increased from 12 billion dollars to 83.4
billion dollars. Of this total, 39 percent, or 31.5 billion dollars, was allocated
for hospital expenditures. The hospital can hardly be viewed as an operation
similar to the corner green grocer which relies on personal relationships and
good will between employer and employees not only to get the job done,
but to assure everyone her or his fair share.

In the so-called good old days, hospital trustees and the medical staff were
responsible for making decisions. With the growth of the health industry and
the infusion of government monies and third-party payments, those responsible
for making decisions now are hospital administrators, trained business types,

lawyers, and computers. The very least one can say about this is that the climate in hospitals has changed.

The businesspeople have taken over and have literally turned hospitals into big business organizations which have the interest of developing profit, and to do this they have created their own bureaucracies. The bureaucracy means a large administrative staff, lots of paper shuffling, computers, and more and more equipment in order to demonstrate that this autonomous entity can function and compete with other institutions. These remarks are not intended to only criticize hospitals, rather they point out the contextual realities in which most nurses function. Given the basic structure of the health care system and the free enterprise system within which hospitals function, these vast changes may be viewed as a natural occurrence. Health and health care for all citizens except the poor and the elderly at present are commodities to be bought and sold in the market place.

Any big business has to find methods of cutting corners. In addition to the quality of the care given, hospitals must consider ways and means of making their operation more efficient. Efficiency of this type can interfere with the quality of the care given. It seems reasonable to assume that nurses necessarily suffer in this kind of environment because health care is comingled with business considerations. Hospitals have not been magnanimous in volunteering to undertake actions to improve the status of nurses but, in my opinion, continue to impose on them low salaries, poor working conditions, and a multitude of other good business practices, since all this saves the hospitals money. The hospital training programs for RNs also provide many cheap workers for the hospitals in the name of education. To a very large extent, nurses in the past have accepted these conditions and, indeed, many still do. Perhaps the press of events in both the nursing profession and in society at large will begin to change this situation for the better.

As an example of some of these problems, in a recent survey conducted with a sample of 10,000 nurses throughout the country, 3,800 said that they would not want to be patients in the hospitals where they worked. Not only did these findings raise serious questions about the quality of hospital care, but they also shocked some leaders of the nations's hospital industry. Specifically, the survey reported that 18 percent of the respondents said that they knew of deaths caused by doctors. Four percent of these nurses reported that they themselves had made mistakes which they believed had led to a patient's death. These findings raise a host of questions regarding the ethical issues in these situations.

One typical situation reported by a nurse told of a shortage of nursing personnel on the evening shift in the intensive care unit where the nurse had responsibility for six patients on ventilators in three separate rooms. This nurse spent about fifteen minutes with one patient who was hemorrhaging and then returned to another room where the patient had accidentally disconnected himself from the machine, arrested, and died. This incident raised the question of human resources and staffing in an area where, by definition, critically ill patients require close attention.

The Nursing Workforce

Three overriding characteristics of the nursing labor force do not differ from most other non-physician hospital employees. Nursing is composed predominantly of women, is highly stratified, and, as already mentioned, most nursing care takes place in large institutional settings. In addition, the nursing labor force as a whole is heavily concentrated, as far as educational credentials go, at the lower degree levels. To emphasize this last point, in 1972, of 778,470 employed registered nurses in the United States, 70.5 percent has less than a B.A. or B.S. degree since they had trained at a hospital school; 14.3 percent had attained a bachelor's degree; 3.2 percent held a master's degree; and 0.2 percent held a doctorate.

With regards to salaries, when educational credentials, skills, and responsibilities are taken into consideration, nursing workers in general receive poor pay relative to other American occupational groups. According to the United States Census Bureau, in 1970, secondary school teachers, social and recreation workers, elementary school and kindergarten teachers made higher salaries than registered nurses did.

In sum, although some nurses at the top of the nursing hierarchy in hospitals and schools of nursing are relatively well paid, at least for women, and have a fair amount of control over the day-to-day work process, the vast majority of nursing workers receive relatively low wages and have little, if any, formal control over the use of their own labor or the product of their labor.

Interacting Variables

With the increasing concentration of registered nurses in large-scale work settings, there is opportunity for better conditions for worker organizations and action. The service nature of the health care industry makes it difficult to carry mechanization or organization of this industry too far, according to some experts. One of the factors impeding organization of the nursing workforce is the nurses' own self-image as women and their self-image as professionals. Women entering nursing in the recent past tended to have a traditional view of the female role. This is to say that nursing was not seen as a career, but as insurance against that day when, as wife and mother, the woman might have to return to the work force.

A labor force composed mostly of women can be hired more cheaply than one composed mostly of men, even though there has been a social movement as well as legal action to attempt to remedy this situation. Women are believed to be dedicated to service and not self-interest, although more and more of them have head-of-household status. Women are expected to drop out of the labor force to raise families, thus obviating the need for promotions or increased pay for seniority. Their fringe benefits and retirement plans tend to be woefully inadequate. In addition, women are viewed as safe because they do not threaten physicians who, in order to expand their own services and therefore their incomes, must be assured of subordinates who will stay subordinate. Women do not have the social power, that is, access to capital, access to specialized education, freedom from family responsibilities, and respect of political leaders, to become organized competition in the medical marketplace. Furthermore, any discussion of women in the labor force must take into account that few occupations have been open to women. The United States census lists eighty major occupational categories and also indicates that in 1970 seven of these categories contained 43 percent of all women workers. The low pay for high skills found in health services is only low compared to white men's opportunities elsewhere. From the point of view of women, the pay is relatively good. Health services have a sex hierarchy as well as an occupational hierarchy. The decision makers are almost entirely male and the workers almost entirely female.

The nursing profession has escaped total control only by repeated self-conscious determination to be an independent profession, yet organized nursing has far less power in the health service industry than one would expect of an occupation comprised of so many workers and one so key to the industry. The American Nurses' Association is often ignored by the health service industry elite and its outside supporters on questions of public policy with respect to health care. Much time and energy over the years has been expended in the fight to be taken seriously and to be included in decisions which will affect both nursing and other aspects of the industry.

Collective Bargaining and the Professional Employee

Since nursing is not taken seriously either at the national level of decision making or institutional level of patient care, nursing has opted to enter into collective bargaining procedures in some states.

Whether nursing is a profession, a semi-profession, or no profession at all, it is important to realize that many nurses perceive themselves as professionals. Once this view has evolved during the professional socialization process, the following basic question regarding collective bargaining arises: Can collective bargaining be reconciled with professional status? In other words, is it ethical to organize?

In the late 1960s several writers acknowledged that white-collar unionization trends were being watched closely by both management and labor, but for some groups such as nurses strike action would seem to be in serious conflict with their ethical standards. In the years since the 1960s, we have seen nursing become increasingly involved in collective bargaining across the entire country.

Nurses have found it increasingly difficult to provide the service they recognize is in the best interests of the client. They recognize that their working environment prevents them from providing even the minimum standard of service acceptable to them as professionals. Acting on their strong feelings of ethical responsibility to both the client and to the employer, such professionals have advised the employer when clients were being short-changed on the quality of professional services which they believe should be, and know could be, rendered. This approach has yielded little or no change, has often yielded no feeling of "real listening by the employer" and no "real two-way communication" between the professional and the employer.

The ethical responsibility to the client along with economic issues has led the professional to the pathway of public information about client jeopardy, and, next, to the pathway of public information in regard to the efforts of the professional to change employer practices. Ethical responsibility to the client as much as economic consideration has led to militant protest against the employer. The number of nurses involved in collective bargaining in all likelihood will continue to grow in the near future. As long as there is a disparity between the professional self-image which nurses have long cultivated and the income they currently receive, there will be widespread dissatisfaction in their ranks. As long as there is disparity between the professional self-image of the role in decision making on patient care and the amount of meaningful participation nurses actually experience, there will also continue to be widespread dissatisfaction in nursing ranks.

One major concern, the strike, tends to receive much attention in any discussion on collective bargaining. With strike illegal in public employment and frowned upon in private hospitals because of the hazard to patients, it is essential that alternative ways for resolving impasses be utilized. Fact finding, conciliation, mediation, and arbitration have been used. In view of the critical nature of nurses' services to the sick, it is essential that legislation, while protecting the right to collective bargaining, provide ways of resolving impasses so that the strike weapon will be unnecessary, if indeed declared lawful.

The emergence of collective bargaining efforts by registered nurses parallels in timing and nature the development of negotiating activity by other professional employees of governments and non-profit institutions. It raises a variety of issues. Among them are the need for an alternative to the strike for an employee group which supplies a vital service, the conflict between professional responsibilities and self-interest as employees, and the lack of legislation to guide labor-management relations.

Nursing Ethics and Collective Bargaining

The Code for Nurses states that the nurse's primary obligation is to the patient.[7] This statement comes from the traditional/professional roots of the nursing profession where the focus is on the immediate individual patient for whom the nurse is responsible for providing care. Collective bargaining and especially the strike are sometimes viewed as social mechanisms which create ethical issues for the individual nurse and for nursing as a profession.

In the ethics of the nurse–patient relationship, such ethical concepts as patient autonomy, beneficence (do good), nonmaleficence (do no harm), veracity (truth-telling), informed consent, and confidentiality become central to our ethical thinking and behavior. The conclusion we reach will be determined by multiple factors including our value system, the way we reason through an ethical dilemma, and the particulars of the situation. For example, the Code for Nurses says: "The nurse acts to safeguard the client and the public when health care and safety are affected by incompetent, unethical, illegal practice of any person." The specific meaning of this sentence depends on the concrete situation. And the possible alternatives for dealing with the issue also depend on the specifics of that situation. In short, ethical and legal (or unethical and illegal) behavior usually occurs in a social context. It is very easy to do the "right" thing in a hypothetical situation, but more difficult in the concreteness of one situation.

In saying that the nurse's first obligation is to the patient, the Code for Nurses focuses on the immediate situation with particular individuals. However, the Code also states that the nurse participates in the profession's efforts to establish and maintain conditions of employment conducive to high quality nursing care. Within the Code this is interpreted to include collective action. The Code specifically says, "Defining and controlling the quality of nursing care provided to the client is most effectively accomplished through collective action."[8]

The ethical questions center on the obligations to the specific patients who happen to be under the care of the nurse at a given time versus the larger issues affecting nursing care both immediately and in the future. Nurses, as professionals, have an obligation both to patients in the immediate situation and to future patients. In addition, most nurses are employees in complex organizations such as hospitals where decisions affecting nursing care are often made by other people. Many considerations come into play in these decisions including money and labor. At times such considerations conflict with the standards of good nursing care. For example, when the hospital administration employs a float nurse who is inadequately prepared to work in the critical care areas of a hospital and assigns her to one of these areas, a problem may be created not only for the float nurse, but also for all the other nurses in that area. This decision can result in potential unsafe nursing practice and, additionally, can divert other nurses from their critically ill patients in order to assist the float nurse. Is it ethical to work in this type of situation if the nurses believe it to be an unsafe one? How can the standards of nursing be maintained in this type of situation? Whether nurses are under contracts obtained by collective bargaining or not, one can easily argue that they have an ethical obligation to seriously question this situation. If the administration is open to such activity then mechanisms can possibly be set up to address the problem of safe nursing care. Based on past experience, however, it can be assumed that some administrations will not be entirely open to such concerns on the part of nurses. This is when collective bargaining activities can provide the type of leverage that nurses need in the complex organization.

But those who oppose collective bargaining for nurses, including some nurses themselves, will argue that in the main nurses enter into collective bargaining for their own benefits such as better salaries and better retirement plans. Collective bargaining then is seen as self-serving and unethical rather than as a professional activity centered on patient care and safety. One can point to the fact that historically nurses have been economically exploited by the health care industry. One can also factually document that some of this exploitation continues today.

It seems reasonable to assume that workers who are appreciated and rewarded for their service tend to be happier in their work and, therefore, provide a higher quality of service. This, of course, is not always the case, but in general an argument can be made for this stance. In this culture the realities of better pay and better working conditions are seen as symbols that indicate that workers are appreciated and taken seriously by the employer.

In many places the Economic and General Welfare program (E and GW) of the professional nurses' association is the bargaining agent for nurses. As bargaining agents, the E and GW personnel are concerned with both working conditions, such as salary and hours of work, and professional issues, such as patient safety.

Having a collective bargaining unit in a hospital does not automatically mean that all contractual agreements between employees and employer will be reached without conflict. When conflict which cannot be ironed out over the bargaining table arises, then, historically, workers have resorted to the strike. This presents numerous ethical issues for all types of workers and especially for those in human service areas such as nursing. Is the strike ever ethically justified? Many would argue that it is not, since such action can create unsafe situations for patients. However, there are mechanisms which have been established by the National Labor Relations Board that lessen, if not eliminate, these unsafe situations.

Many in nursing and labor relations believe that as long as health care is big business with economic gains involved nurses will increasingly enter into collective bargaining. And once that step is taken there may come a time when the strike with all its ethical issues may be viewed as the only option open to nurses. The important thing to keep in mind in these situations is that nurses have the ethical obligation to act responsibly toward the patients who are in their care and to work toward making nursing care better for those patients yet to need services.

Summary

Much of the health care in this country occurs in hospitals which are complex social institutions. The social nature of these institutions and the participants in them create dynamics that can affect the ethical thinking and behavior of nurses who constitute a majority of health care workers.

The Code for Nurses is a useful guide to ethical behavior but cannot easily and specifically address ethical dilemmas that arise when moral claims conflict. In order to deal with the social and professional constraints that they confront in hospitals, some nurses have entered into collective bargaining. Both the structural constraints and collective bargaining have ethical dimensions.

Unionization and collective bargaining have been historically the major mechanism by which numerous groups have protected themselves against the greater power and control of owners and employers. That some greater justice and fairness may now exist in the distribution of benefits and income among groups is due to the fact that they fought hard for just demands using the techniques of collective bargaining. Always, it can be argued, the greater justice of outcomes of these struggles stems from the justice of the demands, not the nature of the collective bargaining process itself. Winning through collective bargaining is not evidence that justice was done.[9]

In the case of nursing, it seems reasonable to argue that nurses can make just demands for better benefits and incomes. Importantly, however, nurses also want to negotiate other facets of their work. In the 1974 San Francisco nurses' strike one issue was critical care nurses' control over who would be allowed to work in these units and their qualifications. It is unfortunate that hospital structure and the nurse's social role in that organization is such that it becomes necessary to bargain for safe patient care.

Recently, several hospitals in different geographical locations negotiated the ANA's Code for Nurses into the contract for their bargaining unit of nurses. This is troubling since such basic ethical principles, although not always easily implemented, transcend specific issues at the bargaining table. The question which needs to be thought through is this: If the Code for Nurses can be negotiated into a contract, can it also be negotiated out the next time the contract must be renegotiated? What can be bargained over at the table are mechanisms to enforce aspects of ethical nursing practice.

Endnotes

1. Marcia Millman, *The Unkindest Cut: Life in the Backrooms of Medicine* (New York: William Morris, 1977).
2. Barney Glazer and Anselm Strauss, *Awareness of Dying* (Chicago: Aldine Press, 1965).
3. G. Simpson, *The Division of Labor* (New York: Free Press, 1960).
4. Fred E. Katz, "Nurses," in *The Semi-Professions and Their Organization,* ed. Amitai Etzion (New York: Free Press, 1960).
5. Simpson, *The Division of Labor.*

6. *Perspectives on the Code for Nurses* (Kansas City: American Nurses' Association, 1978).
7. *Ibid.*
8. *Ibid.*, p. 57.
9. Norman Daniels, "On the Picket Line: Are Doctors' Strikes Ethical?" *The Hastings Center Report,* February 1978, pp. 24–29.

In dealing with the problem of conflicting loyalties and nursing accountability, MacIntyre examines historical and current nurse-physician roles and relationships and concludes that they are not functional in terms of meeting the patients' needs. After arguing that the care-cure distinction of medical and nursing functions is not helpful in solving the dilemma, he prescribes a new function for the nurse as interpreter and offers recommendations for the preparation of the nurse to function adequately in this role.

5

To Whom Is the Nurse Responsible?

Alasdair MacIntyre

The question "To whom is the nurse responsible?" presupposes a prior answer to the question "For what is the nurse responsible?" The difficulty in answering this latter question is a result of the historical definition of nursing. When I speak of "definition" here, I am not talking about the kind of definitions that appear in nursing textbooks; I am talking about the way in which, in practice, this or that activity has been allocated to nursing.

This process of definition through the assigning of activity has a long social history in which each medical and health care role is defined, to a greater or lesser degree, in terms of the others. In the case of nursing the degree of definition in terms of other roles has been large. For a very little consideration makes it clear that nursing has been to a surprising extent defined residually; to the nurse has been allocated whatever has been left over from the often self-defined functions and tasks of the physician and surgeon and the bureaucratically defined tasks of the hospital administrator. That is, "nursing" as a label covers a rag-bag of activities with no underlying real unity. (To say this is in no way to denigrate the importance of the nurse's tasks or role.)

To this the reply will at once be made: surely nursing is well-defined. It is centrally concerned with the *care* of the patient, and *care* is to be contrasted with *cure*. But what I want to maintain is that *care* itself is a residual category, a rag-bag label. If a well-defined notion of care were connected with a well-defined notion of nursing, we should not have the difficulties that we have. We do, of course, often suppose the notion of "care" to be well-defined because we contrast it with what we take to be a well-defined notion of "cure;" we are often dominated by a belief that the physician or surgeon is engaged in identifying a well-defined set of symptoms which warrant a well-defined therapeutic intervention the results of which can be observed. "Care" by contrast refers to the background activities, to the sustaining of the patient during the period of the therapeutic intervention. The assumption embodied in this distinction is that if we were to catalog everything that was done to, for, and with the patient during a stay in hospital, we should in general be able to distinguish those episodes that were therapeutic interventions from those that were not. But this assumption is false. It is, of course, very easy to recognize certain classes of therapeutic intervention—the administration of an antibiotic, for example, or the removal of an appendix. But we know that the confidence of a physician or a surgeon in the treatment that he or she is administering is a statistically significant factor in the success of certain chemical and even surgical therapies. We know that "waiting to see what will happen" is one way, and possibly even the best way, to cure certain illnesses; and we know that stress, sleeplessness, and isolation are all factors that can inhibit cure. Given such knowledge, what can we rule out as therapeutic intervention and identify with any certainty as " mere" care?

Some analytical philosophers of medicine—John Ladd, for example—have produced interesting catalogs of conceptual differences between "cure" and "care." Ladd has pointed out that cure has as its object a disease or a disorder, care a person; that cure has a terminus, a point at which it is complete, but care does not—and so on. I do not want to seem to underestimate the importance of deepening our understanding of such distinctions. Ignoring them may always be a source of damaging confusion. But I am afraid that laying too much emphasis upon genuine conceptual distinctions may lead us to overrate the practical importance of the distinction between "cure" and "care." Or rather, it may lead us to ignore the fact that the social importance of this distinction has lain in its ideological function of concealing the lack of intellectual justification for the established division of labor and the conventional hierarchies of the medical and health care world.

At the ideological level we have all learned somehow or other that physicians and surgeons cure, nurses care. But what utterances such as this help to conceal from us is that in practice "cure" is partly defined in terms of "what physicians and surgeons do" and "care" in terms of "what nurses do"—and not the other way around. Ideology inverts reality. Thus in reality what is handed over to the category of "care" is what is left over from the category of "cure;" and both categories and functions are in fact secondary to roles.

The roles of nurse, of physician or surgeon, and of patient are, as I suggested at the outset, to some degree mutually interdefinable. If, as I have now suggested, those mutually interlocking definitions have at the level of theory a vacuous character, if the functions in terms of which the different roles are distinguished are ill-defined, what about the level of practice? Does the emptiness of manifest function point to something concealed, to some latent function? It is important at this point to look at the part that the patient plays in the definition of the relationship of the nurse to the physician or surgeon. It is because the patient is conceived of as having two distinct kinds of needs, a need for "cure" and a need for "care," that the nurse's role can be conceptualized in the way that it has been. But this classification is imposed on the patient by an interpretation of the patient's situation and utterances which is an artifact of the physicians' and surgeons' methods and training. What the patient him- or herself brings to the medical situation is an assorted collection of complaints whose unity is negative: they all belong to the category of *what seems to detract from my well-being or health.* The concept of health is sometimes held to be vague; but it is important not to confuse indeterminacy with confusion. The patient's concept of his or her own health—like many other socially important concepts—will characteristically be open-textured and not fully specifiable in explicit terms. What the patient does or says to express that concept and thereby to limit or define his or her statements of complaint will always, therefore, require interpretation by somebody. The interpretation that the patients' actions and utterances generally and characteristically receive, the interpretation that is crucial for deciding how those actions and utterances are to be evaluated and responded to during the diagnostic and clinical process, is of course that produced by physicians or surgeons. But physicians and surgeons are people who have been systematically taught not to speak the language of the patient any longer. They have been indoctrinated into and taught to speak the language of a theory of symptoms and diseases underlying which there is a concept of health by no means identical with that of the patient. Hence the physician or surgeon brings to the encounter with the patient an often deeply sympathetic, but equally often alien understanding of the patient. It is not going too far to say that the encounter of doctor with patient is characteristically to some degree the encounter of two alien cultures. This is as characteristically unrecognized, although certain features of the task of interpretation do find their place within accounts of diagnostic and clinical judgment. Nonetheless, the task of interpretation extends far beyond what is customarily allocated to it in accounts of such judgments.

The patient's needs, therefore, do *not* come to us categorized in such a way as to justify the definition of the roles of physician and surgeon or nurse. It is rather once again the other way around; it is because the roles of physician and nurse are related as they are, and because physicians and surgeons correspondingly produce interpretations of the patients' actions and utterances which match the definitions of roles, that the needs of the patient are categorized as they are. It is also true that this categorization of the patient's needs is responsible for the fact that one of the patient's key needs, that for interpretation and for an interpreter, is almost completely concealed from view. Thus, one task of the highest importance remains unassigned altogether. The deficiencies in the definition of the relationship of the role of nurse to that of physician are in part responsible for what is often a deficiency in the practice of medicine. And it is not any rationally defensible view of the medical division of labor which is embodied in the physician–nurse relationship.

What then is it that is embodied in the definition of the physician–nurse role relationship? The answer seems to be twofold: there is a *survival* from a certain phase in the history of medicine and there is a latent function in respect of *power* and *conflict*. The phase of medicine in question is that which runs roughly from 1910 to 1965. It is the phase at the outset of which the medically most important causes of death in the United States were the ten major infectious conditions and at the close of which the medically most important causes of death were and are the three major chronic conditions, heart disease, stroke, and cancer. Patients no longer die of tuberculosis or poliomyelitis; as a result they live long enough to contract heart disease or cancer. It was in this period that the final victory of medicine as a collection of applied sciences appeared assured. To treat a patient was to bring about or inhibit chemical or other changes in tissue in precisely the same way that such changes could be brought about or inhibited by the natural scientist; a patient was a locus for such activity who happened to be lying on a bed instead of on a laboratory bench. The forms of specialization of medicine replicate the specializations of the natural sciences.

From this point of view the subordination of the nurse to the physician was natural and right. Nurse stands to physician as laboratory technician to scientist. Care is a mere substructure for the activities of cure. But with the change in focus of medicine which necessarily follows on the change in the causes of mortality this view of the relationship loses what justification it had. The patient-treatment relationship is now very often long-term; the therapeutic interventions of physician or surgeon are episodes in an extended narrative. The function of both nurse and physician cannot be the same, and the relationship of those functions cannot justifiably remain the same. If it does so remain—as it largely does—then it has to be understood as an unjustified survival, whose maintenance has the effect of preventing the raising of key questions about power, status, and money.

What I have tried to do is to deploy in bare, skeletal outline an argument whose conclusion is threefold: first that the current relationship of nurses to physicians and surgeons purports to be, but is not, functional; second, that philosophical analysis at the conceptual level of such notions as "cure" and "care" may unwittingly operate as an ideological disguise for this lack of function; and, third, that there is a function waiting to be performed which goes unperformed, that of interpreting the patient to the physician and, of course, vice versa. The most obvious person to perform this function is the nurse.

This conception of the nurse as interpreter or translator, as emissary between two cultures, that of the patient and that of the physician and surgeon, is one which receives little or no support from current patterns of nursing education. For it suggests the need for a kind of sensitivity to questions concerning communication of a variety of kinds, to uses of language, to the relationship of body and mind, which have been the concern of philosophy and of literature, subjects that have not loomed large in nursing education. But of course the reformation of nursing education by bringing it into far closer contact with the humanities would have little or no point unless there were also a radical change in the power and status relations of nurse and physician.

This, however, does not mean that we need to wait for such a radical change to make the humanities relevant to nursing education. Indeed a transformation of the humanistic ingredient in nursing education may itself be an important agency in leading to social and political change. For the study of history, of literature, and of philosophy enlarges the practical and the conceptual imagination. These subjects teach us not to be too impressed by the conventions of the present and the recent past. They teach us also how to discover the weaknesses and the deficiencies of the present and thus to identify points at which there is a cogent argument available for redefining roles and relationships. It is one such point—that at which the patient's needs demand interpretation—that I have tried to identify in this paper.

Bandman emphasizes the rights as well as the responsibilities of nurses who function as patients' rights advocates. She takes the position that nurses are responsible to the physician, patient, and the hospital, and that all three are responsible to the nurse for justice toward every person's rights. Discussing the Tuma case in depth, she takes the position that while the nurse does have a right to dissent against prescribed medical treatment in some appropriate instances with recommendations of alternative, accepted medical treatment, she has no right to recommend unscientific alternatives to prescribed medical treatment.

6

Who Will Advocate for the Nurse Advocate?

Elsie L. Bandman

Health care has become big business. It is the nation's third largest industry, largely dominated by the medical profession, and focused mainly on the treatment of illness. One writer characterized the American medical care system

> as a great, impersonal, Hydra-headed technological monster clanking across the landscape gobbling up the Gross National Product and excreting computerized bills, neither curing nor caring, growing two new hospital wings and a cobalt radiation unit for every general practitioner that is lopped off and engineered by greedy villains.[1]

Others characterize "the medical structure . . . as an empire with millions flocking daily to its citadels seeking help. Some seek the pursuit of health and of its priesthood, the physicians, as a religion."[2] Without doubt, the millions who are reputedly flocking to the hospital citadels are doing so precisely because of the enormous growth of technology which offers so many life-saving devices and measures hitherto unimagined.

As a consequence of their complexity, hospitals have become vast bureaucratic technological systems characterized by a hierarchy of responsibility, authority, and status. Services are specialized and systematically divided. Roles are defined as a cluster of expectations and prescribed duties which allow for easy replacement of individuals occupying roles low in the hierarchy, such as

Reprinted with the permission of *RN Magazine*.

those of patient and of nurse. Both roles are seen to have universal characteristics of passivity and compliance. According to Talcott Parsons, the person occupying the sick role is excused from the performance of her or his other roles and not held responsible for her or his incapacities. The individual is obligated to behave appropriately in that role which is to seek medical advice, to permit others to care for her or him, and to want to get well.[3] According to Tryon and Leonard, the question of patient role definition is answered by the professional, in practice, as a very passive role for the patient.[4,5] Willard Gaylin, an eminent psychiatrist, described the patient role in the hospital as one which

> exposes an individual to a condition of passivity and impotence unparalleled in adult life, this side of prison. . . . Hospital regulations are endured by a patient conditioned to seeing his physician as a benevolent father in whose reassuring presence he is prepared to play the role of a child. Beyond this, however, more serious rights are violated under the numbing atmosphere of the same paternalism.[6]

Within Gaylin's protest is suggested what Baziak and Dentan have called the role of the nurse as a handmaiden and fulfiller of orders and the patient as a "symptom-vehicle" for the physician who commands in the name of "we."[7] The authors explain the inappropriate behavior of such physicians and nurses as conditioned by a subculture and its language as one in which "prescriptions are orders, patient's comments "complaints" and patients themselves numbers. . . . [and] in which sick people who come to an institution and take care of themselves are labelled 'cooperative' and those who make demands on the personnel are labelled uncooperative."[8]

Gaylin's analogy of the hospital patient's passivity and impotence as like that of a prison is supported in an interview with Connie Williams reported in the *Boston Globe* of December 11, 1977. As a lobbyist for a group actively supporting the passage of the patient's rights measure in the Massachusetts legislature, she likened the patient's rights to a person's rights as a suspect. "When a person is picked up for his crime his rights must be read to him. They are inherent rights which belong to every American under the Bill of Rights."[9] Gaylin supports Williams' contention that the *Statement of a Patient's Bill of Rights* is simply a restatement of basic human rights contained in the American *Bill of Rights.*

> The objection to this well-intended though timid document is that it perpetuates the very paternalism that precipitated the abuse . . . it creates the impression that the hospital is "granting" these rights to the patient. The hospital has no power to grant these rights. They were vested in the patient to begin with. If the rights have been violated, they have been violated by the hospital and its hirelings. . . . In effect, all that the document does is return to the patient, with an air of largesse, some of the

rights hospitals have previously stolen from him. It is the thief lecturing his victim on self-protection.[10]

If the statements made by Willard Gaylin and Connie Williams have any validity, then the reported opposition to the passage of the *Patient's Bill of Rights* by the Massachusetts Medical Society and the teaching hospitals is of no surprise.[11] The fight for patient's rights has reportedly been waged for nineteen years and its present passage is still not assured, with or without the amendment by the Medical Society requiring that only "reasonable requests" be answered.[12]

What is the basis for this amount of opposition to a document which has been characterized as "timid" and "well-intentioned?"[13] The basic opposition may stem from its departure from the authoritarian and benevolent paternalistic model of the omnipotent, omniscient physician–patient relationship toward a contractual or collegial model in which the consumer occupies a position of autonomy and self-determination regarding the treatment of his or her own body. In these last two models, the final decisions are the consumer's, based upon principles of full disclosure and informed consent. Moreover, if the collegial model were selected and implemented, it would require the physician to treat the nurse as a colleague, equal but different, with whom the physician would need to collaborate and consult.

The most significant, if half-hearted, movement toward implementing this model has been the American Hospital Association's *Statement on a Patient's Bill of Rights* in those provisions which state the patient's right to

complete current information concerning . . . diagnosis, treatment, and prognosis in terms the patient can be reasonably expected to understand . . . [and] information necessary to give informed consent prior to the start of any procedure and/or treatment . . . the medically significant risks involved, and the probable duration of incapacitation. Where medically significant alternatives for care or treatment exist, or when the patient requests information concerning medical alternatives, the patient has the right to such information.[14]

These statements contain the truth-telling functions of the *Bill* and go to the very core of the relationship between client, physician, nurse, and the institution in which care is given. This document further states that "legal precedent has established that the institution itself also has a responsibility to the patient."[15] Precisely what the institution's responsibility is has not been clarified. An argument might be made that the client has a clear right to know that an error was made in his or her medication, diet, laboratory test, X-ray, or even surgery. Restitution should be made or awards given for support where there is permanent injury to the patient. This would lead to more just hospital policies and practices. At present, poor, aged, and unsophisticated patients are, for the most part, helpless in the impersonal, bureaucratic system. They tend not to know, to understand, or to ask what the diagnosis, treatment, prognosis, risks, or alternatives are for them. These patients in particular need a nurse advocate to protect their human rights as patients.

The question who should inform the patient of the diagnosis, treatment, prognosis, and medically significant alternatives, and who, if anyone other than the physician, has the right to inform the patient of non-medical alternatives is the crux of the issue. The *Statement on a Patient's Bill of Rights* declares the function of informing the patient to be the prerogative of the physician based on the recognition that "a personal relationship between the physician and the patient is essential for the provision of proper medical care."[16] The *Statement* goes on to say that it is expected that these rights "will be supported by the hospital on behalf of its patients, as an integral part of the healing process."[17] Who or what constitutes the hospital is not defined. A dictionary definition of the term "organization" includes an administrative and functional structure as well as the personnel of such a structure.[18] Does this definition imply that nursing personnel are simply an extension of the functional structure of the hospital without an independent role and that the personal relationship exists only between the physicians and the patient?

If so, then the indispensable role of nursing in providing twenty-four-hour daily continuous personal patient care is denied. But it cannot be denied, since, among all health professionals, nursing is responsible both for coordinating the twenty-four-hour functions of care and for the delegated medical functions of the physician. Consequently, it is nursing, rather than the medical staff, that occupies the key personal position as a consequence of prolonged, continuous, intimate contact with the patient, his or her anxieties and need for information.

The National League for Nursing in its recent statement on *Nursing's Role in Patient's Rights* takes the position that "in many cases, nurses can directly involve themselves in assuring specific rights; in others, they can make their influence felt indirectly."[19] The document clearly states which patient's rights nurses have a responsibility to uphold. They are the right to quality care which is accessible; the right to non-discriminatory, courteous, equitable, and individualized health care; the right to privacy and confidentiality; the right to refuse treatment, medications, and participation in research and experimentation.[20] Most central to this paper is that right which provides for the patients' right "to information about their diagnosis, prognosis, and treatment—including alternatives and care and risks involved—in terms they and their families can readily understand, so that they can give their informed consent."[21] The League document acknowledges that the patient receives direct care from a health team with implications for a variety of people; nevertheless, it states that "in many cases, nurses can directly involve themselves in assuring specific rights. . . ."[22] This very general directive leaves a wide margin for individual discretion. Does it imply, for example, that a nurse like Jolene Tuma of Idaho has the right to recommend "alternate methods of treatment for cancer, namely, the natural approach such as nutrition, herbs, touch therapy, and Laetrile?"[23] Despite Ms. Tuma's appeal to the *Statement on a Patient's Bill of Rights,* the Idaho Nurse Practice Law, and the American Nurses' Association *Code for Nurses* in her defense, Ms. Tuma's license was suspended by the Idaho Board of Nursing and the decision supported by the Idaho State Nurses' Association. Several points can be made about this case. Was Ms. Tuma safeguarding the patient's rights to know alternatives or was she interfering with the "physician's course of treatment as charged?"[24] Is the "personal relationship between the physician and the patient . . . essential for the provision of proper medical care"[25] the only relationship necessary for the provision of proper medical care? Or was Ms. Tuma's recommendation, unscientific and unverified, her participation in the provision of medical care?

The evidence at the hearing supported the charge of interference with the physician's course of treatment, since the administration of the chemotherapeutic agents was delayed by some twelve hours while the patient and her family considered the natural approaches to treatment of cancer. However, refusal of treatment is the patient's right to the extent permitted by law along with information concerning the consequences of the act.[26] The second point, namely that the "personal relationship between the physician and the patient is essential for the provision of medical care"[27] is clearly documented in the American Hospital Association's *Statement on a Patient's Bill of Rights.* Several interpretations of this statement in relation to the Idaho Board of Nursing's decision are possible. One line of reasoning maintains that the physician–patient relationship is primary and exclusive, concerned only with medical care and that the proposal of non-medical alternatives interfered with the delivery of medical care. This point is made in the *Statement on a Patient's Bill of Rights.* "Where *medically* significant alternatives for care or treatment exist, or when the patient requests information concerning *medical* alternatives, the patient has the right to such information."[28]

This provision, specifically the words "medically significant," is the nub of the Tuma case. Since Ms. Tuma "testified that she had a collegial relationship with the physician and that teamwork between nurses and physicians was important"[29] she could have informed the physician in charge of the patient's request for alternatives to medical treatment and her compliance with this need for information concerning natural approaches to the treatment of cancer. The National League for Nursing's statement says simply that "Patients have the right to information about their diagnosis, prognosis, and treatment—including alternatives to care and risks involved—in terms they and their families can readily understand, so that they can give their informed consent."[30]

Jolene Tuma did exactly that and no more. This statement does not limit the alternatives to medical choices. The alternatives Ms. Tuma proposed, namely nutrition, herbs, touch therapy, and Laetrile are widely considered to be non-medical measures unverified by scientific procedures and, therefore, not alternatives to chemotherapy, surgery, or radiation. Until such time as research money is allocated to support trials and investigations of natural approaches to the treatment of cancer, its advocates are placed in the same position as is an astrologer or one who reads tea leaves for guidance in life's problems. Belief in the usefulness of Laetrile as treatment of cancer is not considered enough for knowing whether or not it is so. The term "knowing" rests on the ability to justify or back up the belief in an appropriate manner.[31] For example, Laetrile has been extensively tested under rigorous experimental conditions on victims of cancer and found to be both useless for cancer and dangerous as well.[32] Standards of judgment are involved and these are evaluated. All evidence is a matter of public record in order that it may be tested again for its evidential adequacy.[33]

The point must now be raised concerning the congruence between the nurse's values and the organization from which she seeks employment. If the nurse accepts employment and maintains affiliation with a medical community which abides by scientific rules of methodology and evidence, then is not that nurse obligated to practice by evidential standards of judgment? According to this view, the nurse patient advocate has no more right to recommend Laetrile than does an advocate of free speech to cry "fire" in a crowded theater when there isn't one. In this view, Ms. Tuma's recommendation was not a bona fide medical alternative as are aspirin, codeine, demerol, and morphine as interchangeable analgesics which nurses commonly recommend both to patients and to physicians as appropriate to the patient's state of pain. Instead, her recommendation was completely outside the domain of empirical medicine, one which was tried and found useless.

What of the nurse's right to dissent and to advocate medical alternatives to medical treatment? One view believes that the nurse has that right, based on professional credentials which rest on the nurse's demonstration of knowledge of nursing and of allied sciences which include some knowledge of medical principles and practices. The present movement toward primary care practitioners in nursing is an example of the trend toward incorporating what was formerly believed to be the exclusive prerogative of the physician, namely a physical assessment and history, into nursing practice. Scheffler, a philosopher, defines the relation of belief and experience to knowledge.

> Attributions of knowledge are not . . . simply descriptive of bodies of lore or types of experience; they express our standards, ideals, and tastes as to scope and proper conduct of the cognitive arts. They reflect . . . our conceptions of truth and evidence, our estimates of the possibilities of secure belief, our preference among alternative strategies of investigation. . . . To learn something significant about the world, we must do more than operate logically upon basic truths that appear to us self-evident, and we must go beyond reasonable generalization of observed phenomenal patterns in our past experience. . . . Thought provides hypothetical ideas in response to the problem . . . These hypothetical ideas are tested in action; using them as instruments for controlled operations

upon nature . . . Some raise expectations that are not fulfilled by experimental outcomes, others accurately foretell the responses of nature. In Dewey's words, the process is one of trying and undergoing—trying an idea in practice and learning from the consequences undergone as a result of such a trial.[34]

The problem put forth by Ms. Tuma is the treatment of cancer to which she responded by suggesting an unconfirmed alternative in the form of Laetrile and other unverified alternatives in the guise of nutrition, herbs, and touch therapy without seemingly informing the patient and the family that these were unverified alternatives to medical procedures. What else could she have advocated to the patient? She could have informed the patient of her right to information about and exploration of her diagnosis, treatment, risks, and the alternatives. She could have notified the physician of the patient's request for non-medical alternatives and the extent of her participation in meeting the patient's need for information in order to arrive at a fully informed decision. She should have been unequivocal in her statements that these were not only unverified alternatives but that there is documented evidence that Laetrile is both useless and harmful. She can and should inform the patient of her or his right to self-determination in all matters affecting his or her own body. She can inform the patient of her right to refuse treatment, medications, or further hospitalization. She can do all of this with confidence and freedom from jeopardy if there is either a law in the state or an institutional policy which supports the *Patient's Bill of Rights*.

Above all, if the nurse accepts Virginia Henderson's goal of professional nursing which is to "substitute for what the patient lacks in physical strength, will or knowledge to make him complete, whole or independent,"[35] then the nurse advocate must assist the patient in securing knowledge from the physician regarding medical treatment. If the patient is unwilling or unable to do so, then the nurse should, in this view, communicate the deficits in the patient's knowledge and attendant doubts to the physician so that the patient may give fully informed consent to medical treatment. As the physician's field of knowledge does not encompass nursing, so does the nurse's field of knowledge not encompass medicine. There is obvious, growing, and unavoidable overlap of the disciplines and questions of territoriality may become critical in some situations. There are, however, areas of freedom and areas of negotiation where the nurse's assessment of the patient's response to illness and treatment are critical factors requiring nurse advocacy. It is in these areas that nursing advocacy may achieve its potential in supporting patient's rights. Both nursing organizations have pointed to the fact of the burden for upholding patient's rights as falling on the shoulders of the individuals who provide their care.[36,37]

What then is the effect of institutional policies and procedures on the role of the nurse as patient advocate? The view here is that if the nurse sees herself as the defender of the patient's rights, she can still function effectively as a hospital employee because in no sense is she the total and only patient advocate. There are obvious courts of appeal for both patient and nurse. There are other members of the health care team, the hospital supervisory and administrative hierarchy, the family, the clergy, and, ultimately, the courts. It may well be that this kind of validation may have been of help to Ms. Tuma in resolving the situation in which she found herself.

In her paper on the institutional barriers that stand in the way of the implementation of the patient's rights or the nurses' rights, Catherine Murphy contends that the nurse is necessarily subordinate to the authority of the institution which like any good bureaucracy has utilitarian goals of the greatest good for the greatest number. This means that the patient's individual rights must be sacrificed for the greatest good of all the other patients.[38]

At this point, I must take exception. As Bertram and Elsie Bandman point out in their paper, "there are justifiable limits on a patient's liberty, privacy, self-determination and capacity to control what happens . . ."[39] There are grounds for justified interference with one's liberty both for one's own interests as well as the good of others. One may have to be restrained from taking heroin, from otherwise unknowingly harming oneself by taking medically inadvisable forms of treatment or by failing to prolong one's life where the evidence may well warrant doing so. "Regarding justified interferences with one's liberty for the good of others, one is restrained from spitting on the streets, speeding on the highways or . . . spreading contagious diseases."[40] Hospital patients must be restrained from smoking in rooms where oxygen or other combustible gases are running, interfering with the rest or the privacy of others by engaging in sexual intercourse, or drinking and partying in hospitals caring for severely ill patients. Above all, patients must be kept from harming or destroying themselves either inadvertently or deliberately. As Bertram and Elsie Bandman point out

> freedom and autonomy are precious but they may not be the only virtue associated with rights. Freedom . . . has limits in the form of rational constraints on what a person may do to others. . . . There is something to be said for connecting one's rights . . . to at least knowing . . . what is in one's interests . . . If the patient too frequently does not know what is best for her or his own interest and what is in the interest of others, there may be reason to question the lack of limits . . . and in particular to question the connection between a patient's right and a patient's freedom.[41]

A further source of conflict for the nurse advocate in a hospital is seen by Catherine Murphy as the dilemma of responsibility. "To whom is the nurse responsible: the patient, the hospital, or the physician?"[42] She sees, in Katz's words, the nurse as both a sponge and a buffer between the professional and the layperson and actively engaged in concealing medical or nursing errors which may adversely affect the reputation of the hospital and the physician. I view these roles and many of the limits on nursing as self-imposed. Nursing has participated in supporting the status quo of the bureaucratic hierarchy of the hospital to a large degree. Too many nurses have been willing partners in the nurse-doctor game in which the nurse advances information or correction to a physician in a way which makes him look good and minimizes her contribution. In general, a neutral or passive stance for nurses has netted various secondary gains, such as administrative upward mobility, social relations otherwise unattainable, or abdication of the need for accountability in nursing. Luther Christman has publicly pointed to the enormous difficulty of identifying the source of nursing errors in hospitals due to the successful process of obfuscation and failure to accept accountability in nursing practice. This is supported by Dr. Murphy's research which fully documents the generalization that "the moral reasoning, the value orientation and role performance of an individual are affected by the moral atmosphere. Socialization of the student nurse has occured mainly in hospitals with the emphasis on bureaucratic goals as incompatible with the individualized needs of patients and the role of the nurse as a locus of autonomy and moral authority."[43] Her research shows most nurses in compliance with the bureaucratic model with the focus on teamwork and team responsibility or as an extension of the physician in the medical model. This model persists because it has some obvious benefits in the form of validation of assumptions and hypotheses, because it has been rewarded and reinforced, and because nursing has been so painfully slow in moving toward an alliance with the health consumer and the general public in a movement for securing patient's rights.

Even as an adherent of the nurse advocate model, the necessary constraints placed upon the individual patient's rights and nurse's rights cannot be ignored. Patients in crisis or emergency are entitled to the complete attention of the necessary nursing, medical, and technical staff while other patients without these serious needs give up their rights to the attention of physicians and nurses at those times. Resources are finite and in any situation of competing claims, the good of the majority must be subordinated to the need of the person in need. Conversely, the less important needs of the individual give way to the priority needs of the group. To meet all individual needs of all patients is simply not feasible in a world where nurses and other health workers must be paid just salaries. Perhaps a just social order is one which includes consideration to the needs of health workers as well as patients. Hospital policies and rules are also necessary since they sometimes simplify what might otherwise be a chaotic situation of autonomous individual nursing practice "according to one's conscience" as Leah Curtin has stated.[44] No one, in my opinion, has the right to practice solely according to his or her moral aptitude, since everyone needs to be checked by the counterbalance of others' evidential judgements and moral sensitivities if bureaucratic violence is to end. I extend this principle to the case of Jolene Tuma who, while practicing as a nurse and a teacher under the

Idaho nurse practice act within a scientific community, informed a patient of three unverified, highly debatable, non-medical alternatives without seemingly informing the patient of their dubious, unverified status all in accordance with her conscience.

Regrettably, no one model supplies all the answers to the issues and dilemmas of patients' and nurses' rights. If patients' rights and nurses' rights are supported without effectively relating to a scientific data base, then immoral situations arise in which the nurse advocates a useless and harmful drug, such as Laetrile, for the treatment of cancer while the patient loses precious treatment time. If the bureaucratic model is totally ignored, the nurse runs the risk of trying to make individual decisions for individual situations without enough concern for the thread of continuity and relationship which ties structures and processes together as in the situation in which the nurse tries by herself to stop police officers from physically assaulting a handcuffed patient in the emergency room of a hospital. This carries me full circle to the answer to Catherine Murphy's question "To whom is the nurse responsible: the patient, the physician or the hospital?"[45] My answer is simply and unequivocally that the nurse is responsible to all three and all three are responsible to the nurse for justice toward every person's rights. The nurse, who in a health maintenance organization in New Jersey assessed a lump in a woman's breast as worthy of a mammography which turned out to be negative and who was then sued by the patient for unnecessary exposure to X-ray needed the support of both the bureaucratic structure and the medical staff. The nurse attempting to stop the physical abuse of the patient at North Central Hospital in the Bronx needed the help of the institution and the physicians. It is now virtually impossible for any one discipline to function in isolation without institutional support and interdisciplinary connections and correction.

As modern technology makes group and team practice inevitable, so must the process of moral decision making involve open and shared processes of decision among health professionals. The patient must be included and so must be the nurse, both on the basis of equal status with all others. Nursing education and practice must enhance the moral sensitivities, ethical choices and actions of nurses. Given this requisite education for moral practice, who will advocate for the nurse advocate who stands alone in opposition to the medical decision? What is the issue in this situation? Is the nurse supporting the patient's wishes or is she supporting the patient's best interests? Is there a necessary contradiction? Not necessarily, since the nurse who like Ms. Tuma believes that the patient's wishes should be considered will probably not permit the same or a different patient to jump out a ten-story window, if preventable. The last possibility may be an impulsive, momentary act of desperation which upon further consideration would be rejected by the patient her- or himself. By comparison, support of the patient's wishes while he or she deliberates the relative merits of traditional medical alternatives of questionable benefit in the case of a dying patient with the doubtful or negative benefits of a non-medical alternative gives the patient the opportunity to decide what is in his or her best interests. The patient's best interests then coalesce with the patient's wishes, and these should be respected by everyone if the patient is both confident and completely informed in terms he or she can understand. Otherwise, the hospital is an unjust system in which the nurse may be viewed as the keeper of the keys and the physician as judge and jury.

This now brings us full circle. A just medical system would not deprive the patient of the right to know both medical and non-medical alternatives, their risks and their predicted consequences. The nursing profession will do its part by educating its students so that they know the difference between their intuition and opinion about a treatment and those treatments which have been empirically verified by methodology and findings open to public scrutiny and scientific criticism. Second, the nursing profession will build a cadre of nursing humanists within a powerful nursing organization. These people will further develop the ethical principles of the *Code for Nurses* which will publicly put us on record as supporting the patient's constitutional right to complete information concerning both medical and non-medical alternatives to treatment, including full documentation for the proven, unproven, and disproven efficacy of each. This is a democratic right.

Third, nursing will stand up alongside the health consumer as an ally and champion of the patient's right to choose freely between her or his sometimes contradictory desires and her or his best interests on the basis of fully informed consent as distinct from either coercion, intuition, or "conscience." Fourth, nursing will educate its students and its practitioners concerning the central tenets of the *Code for Nurses*. These concern not only the patient's right to know about and to receive and to refuse treatment, but the nurse's right to participate or withdraw from situations in which he or she is personally opposed to the delivery of a particular form of health care.[46] Both action and inaction presume accountability which the *Code* defines as "providing an explanation to self, to the client, to the employing agency and to the nursing profession." The *Code* further qualifies accountability by specifying the "interdependent relationship of the nursing and medical professions . . . [requiring] collaboration around the need of the client . . . in . . . joint practice as colleagues . . ."[47]

When nursing acknowledges these principles as necessary conditions for advocacy, it can then support all the nurse advocates of the future to implement their practice with knowledge, sophistication, and finesse. Above all, nurses may then be open supporters of the whole truth, committed to advancing the movement of health care institutions toward their ideal function as centers of justice and human rights in health care delivery along with scientific, comprehensive, and humanistic nursing care and cure.

Endnotes

1. H. J. Geiger, "Who Shall Live?" *The New York Times Book Review,* March 2, 1975.

2. E. L. Bandman and B. Bandman, "Rights in and to Health Care" in *Bio-ethics and Human Rights: A Reader for Health Professionals,* ed. E. L. Bandman and B. Bandman (Boston:Little, Brown, 1978), p. 256.

3. T. Parsons, "Definitions of Health and Illness in the Light of American Values and Social Structure," *Journal of Social Issues* 8 (1952), p. 2.

4. P. A. Tryon and R. C. Leonard, "Giving the Patient an Active Role" in *Social Interaction and Patient Care,* ed. J. K. Skipper and R. C. Leonard (Philadelphia: J. B. Lippincott, 1965), p. 125.

5. R. N. Wilson, "The Social Structure of a General Hospital" in *Social Inter-action and Patient Care,* ed. J. K. Skipper and R. C. Leonard (Philadelphia: J. B. Lippincott, 1965), p. 236.

6. W. Gaylin, "The Patient's Bill of Rights," *The Saturday Review of the Sciences* 1 (March 1973), p. 22.

7. A. T. Baziak and R. K. Dentan, "The Language of the Hospital and Its Effects on the Patient" in *Social Interaction and Patient Care,* ed. J. K. Skipper and R. C. Leonard (Philadelphia: J. B. Lippincott, 1965), p. 273.

8. *Ibid.,* p. 277.

9. "Q & A with Connie Williams: A Bill of Rights for the Patient is Her Con-cern," *Boston Globe,* December 11, 1977.

10. Gaylin, "The Patient's Bill of Rights."

11. "Q & A with Connie Williams."

12. *Ibid.*

13. Gaylin, "The Patient's Bill of Rights."

14. *Statement on a Patient's Bill of Rights,* (Chicago: American Hospital Assoc-iation, 1973), p. 1.

15. *Ibid.*

16. *Ibid.*

17. *Ibid.*

18. *Webster's New Collegiate Dictionary*, s. v. "organization."

19. *Nursing's Role in Patient's Rights,* (New York: National League for Nursing, 1977).

20. *Ibid.*

21. *Ibid.*

22. *Ibid.*

23. J. L. Tuma, "Professional Misconduct?" *Nursing Outlook* 25 (September 1977), p. 546.

24. P. Jory, *Gem State: the RN Newsletter,* (Boise, Idaho: Idaho Nurses' Associ-ation, October, 1976).

25. *Statement on a Patient's Bill of Rights.*

26. *Ibid.*

27. *Ibid.*

28. *Ibid.*

29. E. H. Zungolo, "Right to Inform Bandwagon," *Nursing Outlook* 26 (Feb-ruary 1978), p. 78.

30. *Nursing's Role in Patient's Rights.*

31. I. Scheffler, *Conditions of Knowledge* (Chicago: Scott, Foresman, 1965), p. 55.

32. "Toxicity of Laetrile," *F.D.A. Drug Bulletin* 7 (November-December 1977), p. 26.
33. I. Scheffler, *Conditions of Knowledge.*
34. *Ibid.,* pp. 2–4.
35. Sister C. Roy, *Introduction to Nursing: An Adaptation Model* (Englewood Cliffs, N.J.: Prentice-Hall, 1976), p. 7.
36. *Code for Nurses with Interpretive Statements.*
37. *Nursing's Role in Patient's Rights.*
38. C. Murphy, "Nurse as a Human Rights Advocate: Challenge and Conflict" (Paper given at the conference, Nursing and Human Rights: A Dialogue, at Long Island University, the Brooklyn Center, Brooklyn, N.Y., May 3, 1978).
39. B. Bandman and E. Bandman, "The Nurse's Role on an Interest-Based View of Patient's Rights" in *Nursing: Images and Ideals,* ed. S. Gadow and S. Spicker (New York: Springer, 1980).
40. *Ibid.*
41. *Ibid.*
42. C. Murphy, "Nurse as Human Rights Advocate."
43. *Ibid.*
44. L. Curtin, "Nurses' Rights and Responsibilities" (Paper given at the conference Nursing and Human Rights: a Dialogue at Long Island University, the Brooklyn Center, Brooklyn, N.Y., May 3, 1978).
45. C. Murphy, "Nurse as Human Rights Advocate."
46. *Code for Nurses with Interpretive Statements,* p. 5.
47. *Ibid.,* p. 10.

SECTION

III

The Nurse's Responsibility to the Patient

Ethical dilemmas in health care involve a conflict of rights or claims among individuals. The patient's right to information or his or her right to make decisions about his or her care may at times conflict with the family's rights or the rights of health care workers who are not permitted to practice their professional skills in a manner which they feel promotes the patient's optimum well-being. Prior to the current patients' rights era, health care professionals made all the decisions which they felt were in the patient's best interest because of their supposed knowledge and expertise in matters pertaining to health. The patients' rights movement has markedly affected the way in which ethical decisions are being made in the health care setting. Complex ethical dilemmas continue to challenge society in determining who shall have the right to decide—patient, family, health care professionals, or courts. The authors in this section deal with the topic of patients' rights and the impact of patients' decisions on their families and health care professionals.

Bertram Bandman examines the conceptual problems of defining rights and he suggests that when we pit the rights of one individual against another we misconstrue the notion of rights based on justice. Healey deals with the problems of developing, implementing, and ensuring a patients' bill of rights and he argues that while nurses ought to be actively involved in protecting patients' rights, they should not be the formal patient advocate in the health care system. Orgel deals with the dilemma of the patient's right to know about her or his condition when the physician decides to withhold the truth. Noting that moral judgments are social, contextual judgments, he deals with the problems of power relationships between nurses and physicians and maintains that power relations are ethically illegitimate. The section closes with Aroskar discussing the conflict of the patient's self-determination as the ultimate value versus the interests of a community of caring which involves the patient as well as those affected by the decision.

Tracing the concept of rights back to Greek civilization in about 800 B. C., Bandman deals with the language of rights and the conceptual problems in defining rights. He argues that the appropriate use of rights is to promote harmony and not to promote adversarial types of relationships. For Bandman, in the context of health care, rights imply harmoniously accepted responsibilities for the patient as an individual as well as for the community as a whole. The notion of rights as an expression of harmony, equality, and respect for everyone's share makes rights in conflict a contradiction.

7

An Alternative View of Patients' and Nurses' Rights

Bertram Bandman

Introduction

We seem to live in a society of rights in conflict, as Elsie Bandman suggests. One example is the by now celebrated case of Ms. Jolene L. Tuma who on March 4, 1976 recommended laetrile to her patient Ms. Grace Wahlstrom without consulting the physician Dr. Patrick Desmond. Questions arise: Did Ms. Wahlstrom's rights as a patient include the right to be fully informed of all alternatives to established medical therapy? Did Ms. Tuma, the nurse and supervising teacher, have a right to recommend laetrile? It seems that in recommending laetrile, Ms. Tuma interfered with Dr. Desmond's treatment of Ms. Wahlstrom. Whether, by interfering with Dr. Desmond's treatment, Ms. Tuma violated Ms. Wahlstrom's health care rights as a patient is yet more serious, especially if interference resulted in harming Ms. Wahlstrom. Issues concerning Ms. Tuma's rights and duties, whether she was morally justified or not and whose rights were violated starkly arise in this case.*

In a conflict of rights between the patient and the physician, the nurse or family members, hospital authorities, and other interested parties, it is not always clear how conflicts of rights of this kind are to be settled.

Other deeper questions may arise: If rights are increasingly in conflict, is there something basically wrong with the language of rights? Do we need another concept?

In this vein several scholars have recently criticized the very concept of rights and its widespread use. Scholars such as Michel Villey, Martin Golding, and others contend that rights are a modern, early enlightenment concept, dating to approximately 1300 and that a society without rights where all these questions about conflicts of rights don't arise at all could conceivably be better than ours.

In addition to raising the above practical questions about how to resolve conflicts of rights, I'd like to propose in this paper that there is reason to believe that rights are not a modern concept, that the early Greeks as far back as 800 B.C. or even earlier had notions that operated very much like our concept of rights, only without some of the drawbacks that our modern concept of rights has acquired, drawbacks that seriously undermine the very real nature and significance of rights. I'd like to suggest, furthermore, that we have reason to again strengthen rights following the example of our Greek and Roman predecessors rather than repudiate rights; and that returning to the Greeks and Romans will help us in re-evaluating cases like that of Ms. Tuma.

Golding's and Villey's Modernity Thesis

First, a brief account of the modernity thesis. To Golding and to Villey rights are a modern concept that dates to Ockham (1280/90–1349). These scholars account for our rights approximately as follows. Around 1320 Ockham identified rights as powers, some of which "conform to right reason" (natural rights).[1] It seems that out of the rights developed by Ockham and later by Locke, according to this account, the first kinds of rights were associated with one's liberty and the duty of others not to interfere in one's sphere of privacy or autonomy. These have come to be known as "option rights."[2]

Over the last century and a half, according to this account, a new kind of right has emerged, the right of powerless groups and persons to be helped. These newer rights are known as "welfare rights"[3] or "subsistence rights."[4] On this view of extended rights, everyone alive has a right to food, clothing, shelter, education, maternity benefits, health care, and a lifetime job with paid periodic holidays. Understandably some critics, like Maurice Cranston and Charles Fried, are scornful of these rights and regard them as frivolous. And some critics of the older option rights, like Golding, point to the excesses of *laissez faire* practices associated with these older rights.

Against the older option rights there is the criticism that a few people can no longer be protected in the right to their freedom without limits imposed on their freedom in an overcrowded world. Regarding the newer welfare rights, there seems to be a danger that with too many people's needs for food, clothing, shelter, and medicine, not all of which can be met, such rights get to be too *thin* to be rights that can be effectively held by anyone. There just isn't enough to go around to provide for such rights. Between either or both of these rights there seems to be no shortage of rights in conflict.

The upshot of the Golding-Villey historical thesis is that if one accepts pre-modern societies as good, then it is possible to have a society without rights and possibly even one that by not having rights is morally preferable to ours. In such a society, neither a patient nor a physician nor a nurse nor family members nor hospital authorities nor the community would argue about rights. Some people including scholars such as Golding would, I gather, argue that such a society is better than ours which generates undesirable conflicts of rights. In a society without rights, the question of Ms. Tuma's rights or of Ms. Wahlstrom's or Dr. Desmond's or Ms. Wahlstrom's family members' rights or the rights of hospital authorities is a question that would never arise. And questions about the resulting conflicts between their rights (with all the acrimonial, adversarial ill-feelings and worsening human relations) are questions that would never arise. For in a society without rights, relations of trust and confidence and compassion between patient and physician could again be revived to what these were like in Greek, Hebraic, Roman, and early medieval times.

An Alternative View of Rights in Greek Antiquity

Evidence against the Modernity Thesis

The evidence, however, does not seem to be so clearly in favor of the Villey-Golding historical hypothesis, even though there are important scholars, such as H. S. Maine,[5] H. F. Jolowicz,[6] and W. W. Buckland,[7] who support the Villey-Golding view. There are, however, other scholars such as Alan Gewirth, along with celebrated Greek and Roman historical and legal scholars such as M. Ostwald,[8] A. H. Adkins,[9] A. W. Jones,[10] and G. Vlastos,[11] who support the notion that if the Greeks did not have an exact word "rights," or if the Greeks did not have an explicit concept of rights, they nevertheless had a notion which was the forerunner of our more developed concept of rights.

According to some scholars, there are no rights in Plato's works. Let's however consider one dialogue, *Euthyphro*.[12] Euthyphro charges his father with impiety for murdering his slave who in a brawl, in turn, murdered another farm hand. Perhaps no rights are explicitly appealed to by Euthyphro. But he does go to court to charge his father with murdering a slave. Did the slave have no rights to life, even as a slave?

Words like *moira*,[13] *eunomia, homonoia, isonomia*,[14] *dike*, and others like these were used. Were these not perhaps the predecessors of our rights, pre-rights words, words that conceivably did the work of rights?[15] As a rose by any other name is still a rose, so a right by any other name is still a right.

I want to go on to suggest that the Greek view of rights may have been richer than ours, that we not give up rights but look to where our modern view may have gone wrong; and by retracing our steps, revive the essential nature and importance of rights.

My impression is that from a Greek point of view, a fundamental criticism of both option rights and welfare rights is that the option rights to do almost anything one pleases, like owning a gun, advocating laetrile, teaching astrology, or manufacturing harmful products, degenerate into exercises of license and erode rights into powers and special privileges that are unlimited in any concern for others.

Welfare rights are too often merely disguised paternalistic requirements, which Joel Feinberg abusively regards as "mandatory rights." Since such rights abrogate one's freedom to decide, he suggests that these are no rights at all.

Even more serious perhaps, such rights are merely a disguised form of "hand outs," a public charity at best reminiscent of the *noblesse oblige* of the old slave-master relation, only in the name of a disgruntled society, angry at the poor but too ashamed to let them starve.

A Third Kind of Right

If we look at Greek notions which were the forerunners to our ideas of rights, we find, however fragmentary these were, that their emphasis was on such Greek terms as *eunomia,* meaning habituated and internalized order, *homonoia,* meaning internalized sense of harmony, and, the capstone of all and also the origin of Greek democracy, *isonomia,* or access to equal justice, translated by some scholars, such as Ostwald, as or fairly close to "equal rights."[16]

Such rights were not connected to an excessive kind of freedom or privacy but to equal justice. The right to equal shares or to one's due, the right to do the right thing with enough but not excessive discretionary freedom characterizes rights based on justice, where freedom, privacy, and license including excess property and the accompanying attitude of greed drop out. (Note in this connection also later critiques of rights by Hegel, Marx, and Engels.) Also welfare rights are a paltry, barely disguised form of *noblesse oblige,* with often too little to go around and distributed in such a way as to demean the recipients. The right not to starve, while it marks an advance over the contemptuous policy of "let them eat cake," if construed as bare subsistence, is clearly not enough of a right to dignify human beings. To Vlastos "Platonic morality leaves no room for a conception of private life in which one has the right to do what one pleases without thought to social service."[17] And Alan Gewirth writes that "It has long been recognized that assertions of rights are often linked to high valuations of individual liberty; indeed Marx went so far as to say that rights-talk including the French Declaration of the Rights of Man, is essentially egoistic."[18]

My suggestion is that the Greeks renounced what we call liberty-rights, but not claim-rights; for they referred to shares, allotments, or allocations based on a deduction from some prior doctrine of political justice, either democratic or nondemocratic. But however one consequently defined one's share, either on a democratic or nondemocratic basis, one was not to transgress one's share (or "due"). For the Greeks then, if we may interpret their notion of "rights" as shares or allotments,[19] there were no rights without rules.

On this view, our term "rights" may have had a number of related Greek equivalents, including *eunomia* or stability of law based on internally accepted order, *homonoia* meaning harmony or absence of faction, divisiveness, and conflict, and *isonomia* meaning equal shares, equal law, or equal "rights." This became for the early Roman thinker Ulpian "the right to do the right thing," characterizing rights based not on freedom but on justice, where freedom, privacy, and license, including excess property and resulting greed are placed in check. And again the relation to Marx's and Engel's critique of the language of rights bears this explanatory comment: that a possible reason for the omission of rights-talk both in ancient Greece and in Marx's work is that rights were identified with avarice.[20] Rights to at least some thinkers carried a negative emotional connotation; and for some contemporary writers, they still do. On this view, even welfare rights are too impoverished to serve as significant rights.

A reason for the repudiation of rights is that they generate adversarial relations which, in turn, lead to animosities, factions, and public dissension. Perhaps individuals in enlightened societies are in excessive conflict with one another to begin with and use the rhetoric of rights to dignify their role in the struggle for power.

This is not what a Greek political thinker, like Cleasthenes or Pericles, Plato or Aristotle, wanted a concept of rights or a concept virtually like rights to do. The Greek idea, with all the differences among democrats and anti-democrats, was to identify justice as harmony rather than conflict in a community. The very idea of adversarial relations and of advocacy, whether in the Tuma case or some other case, like the *Darling* case (in *Darling* v. *Charleston Comm. Hospital,* 211, N.E.2nd 53, Ill., 1965) would be the deathblow of justice.

Against those who argue that there were no Greek words for and therefore no concept of rights, there were not only terms like *isonomia* but there were also terms like *aisa* and *moira*. At the time of Homer (800–900 B.C.) the word *moira*, while it may have referred to one's death, referred also to one's fate; but *moira* was also used to refer to one's share, or allotment; and it was hubris ever to transgress one's share.[21]

I'd like to suggest that we consider a further kind of right, one that is more faithful to a richer notion of rights than either our modern concept of option rights or our ultra-modern concept of welfare rights, either or both of which are fairly obviously defective. According to Vlastos, "Ulpian adds 'jus' to 'sum' . . . in his famous definition" that "justice is the constant and unremitting will to render to everyone his own."[22] Rights are not unlimited freedoms. Rights in the plural are connected to right and justice rather than to freedom without concern or duty toward others in one's community.

A further kind of right then, but really the only kind worth having, incorporating Greek notions which were the forerunners of rights, involving *eunomia, homonoia, isonomia,* and *moira* (along with *theopolos* or title or contract, along with a notion used by Aristotle *ta allotria* or *ta hautori* where justice is defined as all having their own) is *the equal right to participate in one's commonwealth* or *community*. This is the right to participate in making the rules one lives by, or for short the right to make rules or the right to rule. This right to share in rule-making sets the boundaries which limit both option rights and welfare rights. These rights may be identified as legislative rights.[23]

In such a role, rights do not function to express and exhibit conflicts nor take sides in disputes, but rather to settle disputes. Rights are, after all, designed to justify action. And rights used in endless conflicts become incapable of being appealed to in rationally settling disputes. In this connection, Oliver Wendell Holmes on more than one occasion noted that the function of a judge is to decide in a dispute "who has gained the rights."[24]

On the third view of rights the duties implied by them are harmoniously taken on and accepted. These are rights that entail no advocates since in such a society rights are not used to win conflicts and so no advocates are needed. The real use of rights is to promote harmony, not promote adversarial proceedings.

To put *moira* in the language of rights, which may not be what the word translates to, it would mean that there are responsibilities around one's rights or shares against which one does not trespass. Otherwise, as seems to be quite regularly the case in our society with its modern use of rights, one exercises not rights at all but powers and privileges.

Even if the foregoing account is regarded as an idealized myth which holds in no world or society we recognize, there is a role of rights not accounted for by those who regard rights only in a conflicting role. Rights are also used in this society as well as in tribal societies to settle disputes.[25] When this role of rights is internalized among the members of a society, rights become exercised in reciprocal relationships with responsibilities and tacitly accepted restraints. Joel Feinberg expresses this point well when he says that one who has rights knows when not to exercise them.[26]

Extending his point consists in knowing what one does not have a right to do. Otherwise, one is using rights language to give emotive support to one's drive for power. Although rights include powers, powers to do and to have, rights are not only powers. Rights are not merely emotive forms of power or rhetoric; rights are rationally justified grounds of action. Rights are a social arrangement giving a person a limited, safeguarded power to act or make claims on others in accordance with an appropriate set of (presumptively just) rules or principles.

Application to the Tuma Case

Applying the alternative view of rights, one that transcends option rights and welfare rights, to the Tuma case, if those involved in the Tuma case had a notion of rights, they wouldn't harm one another nor be in conflict. Rights are not in conflict. Rights are an expression of harmony, stability, equality of consideration, and respect for one's share. The Greek notion of justice as *eunomia, homonoia,* and *isonomia,* with each individual's *moira,* share, or equal right, makes "rights in conflict" a contradiction.

In the context of health care, rights imply harmoniously accepted responsibilities not only to patients, hospital authorities, nurses, and physicians. Such rights imply responsibilities toward one's community as a whole. There are no rights outside a simultaneously practiced set of just rules.

Similarly, the physician's or nurse's right to strike or the hospital administrator's right to provide unacceptable health care conditions or the patient's right to abuse health professionals or fellow patients, as well as a health professional's right to recommend a drug such as laetrile against which there is considerable evidence—these are all misconceptions of rights based on justice.

In our society we pit individuals against one another and arm them with rights. In desperate situations we give anyone with an opinion the right to suggest helpless remedies to a dying person. We give the patient the right to be fully informed when there is an absence of information, as there is concerning viable alternatives in desperate situations.

Rights as justified grounds of action involve cognitive considerations. In questioning a right to inform a patient about X (e.g., laetrile), for example, questions of "How do you know X (laetrile) has Y properties?" or "What gives you the right to recommend X?" are questions that are not out of order. The right to inform a patient, accordingly, does not consist in the right to misinform a patient. Informing rather than misinforming a patient involves at least some knowledge. In this sense, the right to inform a patient presupposes appeal or possible appeal to cognitive considerations in answer to challenges of the form: "How do you know X has property Y?" The right to inform, as does any right, implies that one knows the scope as well as limits of such a right. One who acts on the basis of such a right knows not to, and does not, transgress the limits. That is part of the importance of returning to the Greek word *moira* as one's share or due. One who acts by one's rights does not go beyond them if they are real rights, rights that are justified and that are justly distributed.

So, on this view of rights, rights involve the responsibility of not overstepping one's *moira* or share and presuppose that one knows one's share. Knowledge involves evidence and regard for evidence. On such a view of rights, one question about Ms. Tuma then is: Did Ms. Tuma know and tell Ms. Wahlstrom, the patient, the evidence for as well as against laetrile? This would have meant that Ms. Tuma stayed within her rightful and responsible *moira* or share and that her recommendation was based on responsibly believed evidence. In the case before us, Ms. Tuma does not seem to have been instructed on these limits to her right to practice.[27]

A further and final consideration about these rights in application to the Tuma case for us in our culture to consider is that on the Greek view of "rights" or their near synonyms, patients ask too much of health professionals instead of being content to die like the carpenter in Plato's *Republic.* When he can no longer get well he accepts the end of life. Such a patient does not bestir himself or herself or others with frantic and dubious remedies. This passage is worth quoting:

> When a carpenter is ill, I said, he expects to receive from his physician an emetic or a purge or to get rid of his disease by cautery or surgery. If anyone should prescribe a long regimen to him, that he should rest with his head on pillows and all that goes with this, he would soon say that he has no leisure to be ill and that life is no use to him if he must always be concerned with his illness and neglect the task before him. After that he would bid his physician good-bye, resume his usual manner of life, and recover his health. If his body could not tolerate the illness, he would die and escape from his troubles. For such a man to use medicine in this way is thought fitting.[28]

Conclusion

We undoubtedly find conflicts of rights if we view rights either as option rights or as welfare rights, rights which are an outgrowth of the modernity thesis dating from Ockham or Locke. Instead of dropping "rights," however, we might therefore consider another kind of rights, one that makes "rights in conflict" a contradiction, one that makes "either-or" rights, such as the rights of Ms. Tuma or Ms. Wahlstrom or Dr. Desmond no rights at all. For on the Greek view, at least, there are no rights, shares, or allotments in conflict. Perhaps some such thought prompted Plato to come close to banishing all talk of rights. On this view, patients' rights, including Ms. Wahlstrom's, are not in conflict with Dr. Desmond's or Ms. Tuma's nor, in turn, are Ms. Tuma's rights in conflict with Dr. Desmond's. There are no rights in conflict.[29]

To have real rights is not to have rights in conflict. An enriched notion of rights, one that transcends both the mediocre freedoms associated with option rights and the paltry values associated with welfare rights, a notion of rights that gives us the equal right to participate in our commonwealth does not give us reason to banish rights.

Against the view that if there were no word for rights, there couldn't have been a concept of rights, the Greeks had a number of related words, like *eunomia,* meaning order, well-being, and contentment, *homonoia,* meaning harmony or consonance of minds and hearts, *isonomia,* meaning equal justice, *moira* or *aisa,* meaning one's share, *ta haton,* meaning to have or possess (How could one possess without having rights?), and *theopolis,* meaning title or contract.

So, against those who said there was no word and therefore no concept of rights, we can I think profitably repeat the remark commonly attributed to Gertrude Stein that "a rose by any other name is still a rose" and say the same thing about rights, which predate Ockham, going all the way to Homer (800–900 B.C.).

Perhaps to accommodate our time as a concession, and also to recognize that in our world, rights without conflict are a myth, an important truth recognized by Elsie Bandman, we may distinguish between power-rights as they are currently used in the welter of conflicts and idealized rights, rights regarded as ideal types;[30] and leave to others to decide which kind are real rights. Bearing this distinction in mind, we may recognize that bidding farewell to unsavory features of rights is not tantamount to waiving all rights forever.

On behalf of Ms. Wahlstrom, Dr. Desmond, Ms. Tuma, and the rest of us, there are not enough compelling reasons, it seems, to banish rights and look for another concept. Instead, we may set about pruning away the wrongs that grow out of the imitations of rights that are paraded before us in the name of rights.

Endnotes

* I am indebted to E. Bandman's paper "Who Will Advocate for the Nurse Advocate?" Her perceptive comments on the Tuma case were most helpful in the present work. This makes it all the more unfortunate that I reluctantly disagree with her implied view that rights conceptually involve conflict.

For further material on the Tuma case, see *Nursing Outlook* 25, no. 9 (September 1977), "Letters," p. 546 and the "Editorial" by E. P. Lewis "The Right to Inform," p. 561; also *Nursing Outlook* 25, no. 12 (December 1977), "Letters," pp. 738–743; *Nursing Outlook* 26, no. 1 (January 1978), "Letters," pp. 8–9; *Nursing Outlook* 26, no. 2 (February 1978), "Letters," p. 78; *Nursing Outlook* 26, no. 3, "Letters," p. 142–143.

However, for primary material, see *Reporter's Transcript of Proceedings,* L. Johnson, Court Reporter, 561 Fifth Avenue North, Twin Falls, Idaho, 83301, Idaho, "Before the Board of Nursing," State of Idaho, In the Matter of: Jolene Lucille B. Tuma, R.N.," July 8, 1976, "Findings of Fact and Conclusions of Law," pp. 1–7. For verbatim discussion of licensee's rights, see pp. 12, 13, 22, 23, 34, 41. For a discussion of conflicts of rights, see pp. 178–180; and for a discussion of the patient's right to be informed, see pp. 215, 227, 238–239

1. M. Golding, "The Concept of Rights: A Historical Sketch" in *Bioethics and Human Rights,* ed. E. Bandman and B. Bandman, (Boston: Little, Brown, 1978), p. 48.
2. Golding, "The Concept of Rights," pp. 44–50.
3. *Ibid.*
4. See my "Option Rights and Subsistence Rights" in *Bioethics and Human Rights,* ed. E. and B. Bandman (Boston: Little, Brown, 1978), pp. 51–61.
5. H. S. Maine, *Dissertation on Early Law and Custom* (London: John Murray, 1891), pp. 356–366, 389–390.
6. H. F. Jolowicz, *Roman Foundations of Modern Law* (Oxford: Clarendon Press, 1957), pp. 66–67.

7. W. W. Buckland, *A Text-Book of Roman Law from Augustus to Justinian* (Cambridge: University Press, 1963), p. 58; *see also* A. Gewirth, *Reason and Morality* (Chicago: The University of Chicago Press, 1978), pp. 63–70, 95–103, 372–373.

8. M. Ostwald, *Nomos and the Beginnings of Athenian Democracy* (Oxford: Clarendon Press, 1969), pp. 69, 96, 113.

9. A. W. H. Adkins, *Moral Values and Political Behavior in Ancient Greece* (London: Chatto and Windus, 1972), pp. 67–68, 74, 87, 104.

10. J. W. Jones, *The Law and Legal Theory of the Greeks* (Oxford: Clarendon Press, 1956), pp. 16, 26, 55–59, 64, 79, 85–92, 151, 202.

11. G. Vlastos, "Justice and Happiness in the *Republic*," in *Plato: A Collection of Critical Essays*, ed. G. Vlastos (New York: Anchor, 1971), pp. 75–78.

12. Plato, *Euthyphro, Apology, Crito,* ed. R. D. Cumming (New York: Liberal Arts Press, 1948), pp. 1–20. For a more explicit reference to rights, at least according to some translators, see Plato's *Crito*, p. 60. Socrates here takes the role of the state and challenges Crito and others with the question ". . . Do you think your rights are on a level with ours?"

13. *See* W. C. Greene, *Moira: Fate, Good and Evil in Greek Thought* (New York: Harper Torch Books, 1944).

14. *See* Ostwald, *Nomos* and Jones, *Law and Legal Theory.*

15. *See* D. Daube, *Forms of Roman Legislation* (Oxford: Oxford University Press, 1956), pp. 10–13, 21, 22, 56, 100. I am indebted to David Sidorsky for pointing out this reference and also for his notion that on the basis of Daube's reconstruction the Greeks and Roman had, in Sidorsky's terms, "de facto rights." I am also indebted to Juan Cobbarubias for suggesting that the notion of "rights" functioned on a "depth grammar" level. Also, Betty Brout, Associate Editor of *Ethical Society* suggested to me that there couldn't have been a Greek idea of democracy without rights. This work may be called "philosophical excavation."

16. Ostwald, *Nomos,* p. 113. Even if these scholars were mistaken, *see,* for example, Thucydides, *The Peloponnesian War,* ed. J. Finley (New York: Modern Library, 1951), p. 179, where, according to Finley's translation, the Thebans "spoke as follows: 'Our city at that juncture had neither an oligarchical constitution in which all the nobles enjoyed equal rights nor a democracy. . . .'" Thucydides also refers to "the rights of the Peloponnesians" on p. 37. He speaks of "assaults on the rights of the Hellas" p. 38; and then an Athenian is quoted by Thucydides as saying, "Our abatement of our own rights in the contract trials with our allies have gained us the character of being litigous," p. 44. This speech took place in 432 B.C.

17. Vlastos, "Justice and Happiness in the *Republic*," p. 77.

18. Gewirth, *Reason and Morality,* p. 95.

19. I am indebted to my colleague Elinor West for suggesting the terms "allotments" and "re-allotments" as possible Greek near-equivalents to our term "rights."

20. For an excellent account of a defense of rights based on social justice in Marx, *see* C. Gould, *Marx's Social Ontology* (Cambridge, Mass.: MIT Press, 1978), pp. 13, 35, 129, 130, 140, 144–145, 148–149, 159, 160, 161, 171–178, 182–186.

21. Greene, *Moira: Fate, Good and Evil in Greek Thought*, pp. 18–20, 37. *See also* A. W. H. Adkins, *Merit and Responsibility A Study in Greek Values* (Chicago: University of Chicago Press, 1960), pp. 18–21. *Also see* Adkins, *Moral Values and Political Behavior*, p. 19.

22. Vlastos, "Justice and Happiness in the *Republic*," p. 75.

23. For a further elaboration and defense of legislative rights, *see* E. Bandman and B. Bandman, "The Nurse's Role in Protecting the Patient's Right to Live or Die" in *Advances in Nursing Science*, 1979.

24. O. W. Holmes "The Path of the Law," in *Law and Philosophy*, ed. E. A. Kent (New York: Appleton-Century-Crofts, 1971), p. 21.

25. *See* M. Gluckman, *The Judicial Process Among the Barotze of Rhodesia* (Manchester: Manchester University Press, 1955), pp. 35–81, p. 166; also his *Politics, Law and Ritual in Tribal Society* (Oxford: Basil Blackwell, 1965), pp. 36–79.

26. J. Feinberg, "Postscript to the Nature and Value of Rights" in *Bioethics and Human Rights*, ed. E. and B. Bandman, pp. 32–34.

27. *See* Reporter's *Transcript of Proceedings*, pp. 181–233.

28. G. M. A. Grube (ed.) *Plato's Republic* (Indianapolis: Hackett Publishing Co., 1974), p. 75.

29. I recognize that this statement flies in the face of a remark by the hearing officer in the Tuma case. According to the Reporter's *Transcript of Proceedings*, Mr. William R. Snyder says ". . . with respect to the constitutional freedom of speech that the licensee has raised, we are in an area of some conflict between rights, constitutional rights," p. 178. This, however, shows that he accepts the prevalent view of rights, that rights are in conflict, or that there is a difference between the practice of legal rights and the concept of moral rights.

30. Such a distinction may explain the actual practice of rights in conflicts, illustrated in the Tuma case, and reveal also the role of rights in rationally resolving conflicts and disputes. However, without our carefully carving out this precious dispute-settling role of rights—which may account for the pardonable exaggeration in this paper—they would soon lose their rational bite.

*Healey examines the concept of patients' rights and the evolution of the pa-
tients' rights movement. His essay points out the benefits of a well-written
patients' bill of rights and makes suggestions as to the desirable characteristics
of a bill of rights and how the bill should be developed. He concludes by offering suggestions on how to prepare nurses for leadership roles in identifying and
protecting the rights of patients.*

8

Patient Rights and Nursing

Joseph M. Healey

The papers brought together in this volume are an accurate reflection of the many and varied issues faced by the contemporary practitioner of nursing. No longer content to be assigned in the health care process a subordinate role contaminated by the biases of sexism and medicine's professional arrogance, today's nurses are seeking to establish their own professional identities and to obtain recognition of their status as care providers with moral and legal rights and duties. Pellegrino, writing of recent developments involving nurses and physician's assistants, has described the current setting:

> The emergence of the "new health professions" in the last decade constitutes what may well turn out to be one of the most significant changes in the social structure of medicine and nursing. While the full implications are yet to be comprehended, they may hold for patients an importance approaching the feats of biomedical science.
>
> It is already clear that many questions are posed which are fundamental to the future of how medical care is provided. Our traditional notions of the division of labor among physicians and other health professionals, the locus of authority and decision-making, and even the partitioning of resources between curative and curing medicine, have all been brought under new scrutiny.[1]

This is an era in which nursing is challenging itself and the other health professions to look carefully at fundamental issues. It is inevitable that this period of re-examination result in uncertainty about the extent of the provider's legal and moral responsibilities. In part, it is the attempt to identify more clearly and more accurately those responsibilities that has been a major source of the desire for the re-examination. Nonetheless, the uncertainty is disturbing and most are eager to reduce or eliminate it.

In such a setting, there is a temptation to overlook the series of challenges to the exercise of authority by all health care providers which have been made by supporters of the concept of patient rights. The claims by patients that they have rights and deserve to be treated as active participants in the health care process would appear to be quite removed from nursing's re-examination of its professional identity. And yet, to overlook such an important force on the contemporary health care scene would be a major error. It is critically important for nurses to appreciate the importance of the concept of patient rights and to understand the concept's implication for nursing practice and for nursing education. This paper is designed to encourage nurses to develop that appreciation and understanding and to integrate them into a re-examination of their professional role in the health care process. The goal which both nurses and patients seek is to obtain the best health care possible, consistent with the protection of the rights of both patients and providers. This consideration of patient rights and its implications for nursing is, I believe, not a diversion but really a necessary immersion in these issues.

II

In large part, the significance of the concept of patient rights is derived from the fundamental experience of diminished health and from the health care relationships designed to deal with it. We have all experienced, in our own lives and in the lives of those we love, the destructive impact of sickness, illness, or injury. This impact can be so great that we often say of the afflicted person that "he is not himself" or "she is not herself," reflecting the extent to which sickness, illness, or injury affects its victim. Stuart Alsop, in the autobiographical account of his struggle with cancer, describes this reality in a poignant manner:

> There is another reason this book is peculiar. It was all written by me, but it was written by different mes. Part of it was written by a me lying in bed in the leukemia ward at NIH in late July and early August, 1971, waiting to be put into a "laminar flow room," to get chemical treatment which might buy me a year or so of life. Part of it was written by a me released from NIH in August with a question mark for a diagnosis, feeling rotten but not rotten enough to stop writing the column for *Newsweek* which is my chief source of livelihood and my chief reason for being as a journalist. Part of it was written by a me feeling sick unto death in September, and indeed nearer to death than I realized at the time. Part of it was written a few weeks later by a euphoric me suddenly feeling

better than I had for years and confident—or almost confident—of a final cure. And part of it was written by a me—the me now writing—faced with a recrudescence of the mysterious disease and again in fear of an unwilling expedition to that "undiscover'd country from whose bourn no traveller returns."[2]

Eric Cassell has attempted to describe this destructive impact in terms of four losses experienced by the patient: loss of a sense of connectedness to the world; loss of a sense of indestructibility; loss of a sense of omniscience; and loss of a general sense of independence and control.[3] The healthy person is generally an active participant in the flow of life. The sick person loses that sense of flow. Such a person may be confined to bed, at a health care facility or home, and may be prevented from engaging in normal patterns of daily activity. The world seems to revolve around the patient, excluding him or her from participation. Since most of us feel that sickness, illness, and injury are things that only happen to others, when they actually do happen, they force us to acknowledge our sense of vulnerability and personal limitation. Also challenged is the healthy person's assumption that the future will be an orderly succession of predictable events. The unexpected and unwanted intrusion of incapacity through sickness, illness, or injury undermines any such assumption. The person in such a situation experiences a general loss of control over his or her life. Others—physicians, nurses, relatives—exercise control over such varied things as daily activities, eating, and the number of visitors. This feeling of loss of control was well captured in the cartoon that showed the patient in bed eyeing the night stand filled with everything a patient could want—beverages, books, tissues, a radio—all of which, however, were beyond the reach of the patient in bed. The frustration in such a situation is real, as is the overall effect of the powerlessness experienced by the patient.

Recognition of the destructive impact of sickness, illness, or injury has influenced both the goals of the health care provider-patient relationship and the manner in which such goals have been pursued. Bernard Barber has described the traditional structure of this relationship.[4] The provider is superordinate, an authority, even a person to be venerated. The patient is expected to be subordinate, respectful, and deferential. The provider is active, knowledgeable, and secure. The patient is passive, frightened, and dependent. In such a relationship, there exists one primary goal: to return the patient to health. Everything is subordinate to that goal, including respecting the patient's wishes and the patient's rights. Such a conceptualization can undoubtedly be successful in some cases, but the nature of modern health care, with its concentration on preventive medicine on the one hand, and on management of chronic degenerative disease on the other, calls for a rethinking and a reconceptualization of the provider-patient relationship. The traditional relationship, based on notions of paternalistic benevolence, encourages dependence of the patient rather than independence. It may encourage excessive or inappropriate utilization of health care services. The traditional relationship may encourage the patient to accept an erroneous concept of health as a static entity which the practitioner gives to the patient. Though one can be excessive in placing responsibility for health solely in the hands of the patient,[5] it is more accurate to regard health as a process of well-being influenced by health provider, patient, and society, in varying degrees. The traditional relationship also discourages affording patient rights a primary role in the process of seeking health or the return to health.

In part because of the perceived inadequacy of this traditional pattern of the provider–patient relationship, and in part as the result of the collision of a significant number of forces within our society during the past seventy-five years,[6] an alternative, modern conceptualization of the pattern has emerged. This pattern, also described by Barber,[7] is characterized by several distinct aspects. The provider and patient identify themselves as partners in the health care process. The primary goal of the relationship is not simply the return of health, but rather the return of autonomy and independence to the patient. Good health is not simply the responsibility of the provider but of the patient and of society as well. Good health is a process which results in large part from the patient's bio-genetic nature, from decisions a patient makes about his or her life (e.g., diet and exercise), from health care interventions by health care providers, and from social influences (especially environmental). To succeed, such a relationship requires the acceptance of active responsibility by the patient. It also requires mutual respect by the parties for each other.

The patient rights movement is both a source of the emerging conceptualization and a means to implement it. This emerging conceptualization can achieve its goals best when patients assert their rights. In the past, nurses have frequently reinforced the traditional conceptualization and played a role (direct or indirect) in undermining patient rights. There are significant indications, however, that nurses today are rejecting that approach and are eager to become active forces in identifying, protecting, and assisting patients in the assertion of their rights. A major theme of this paper is that this is a desirable shift which should be encouraged. As they engage in the re-examination of nursing in general and the nurse–patient relationship specifically, nurses should be encouraged to reject the traditional dominance model and to accept the emerging partnership model. To do so, nurses need to have an accurate understanding of the rights of patients. More important, nurses need to be committed to the principles that underlie those rights and to the development of mechanisms for the protection of the rights of patients.

III

The patient rights movement is based upon two key principles:

1. A patient is a person who possesses the same rights as a person generally in society;

2. A patient does not surrender any of his/her rights by virtue of becoming sick, injured, or entering a health care facility.

A major challenge facing supporters of patient rights is the careful delineation
of what those rights are and how they can be protected. There is a major role
for nurses to play in assisting in this process.

Examples of the rights which the patient possesses include the following:[8]

1. The right to self-determination (as represented by the doctrine of
   consent to treatment);[9]
2. the right to refuse treatment;[10]
3. the right to have access to information;[11]
4. the right to have information treated as confidential;[12]
5. the right to receive appropriate quality medical care;[13]
6. the right to terminate a provider–patient relationship.[14]

The best known formulation of these rights is the American Hospital Association Bill of Rights:*

The American Hospital Association presents a Patient's Bill of Rights with
the expectation that observance of these rights will contribute to more
effective patient care and greater satisfaction for the patient, his physician, and the hospital organization. Further, the Association presents
these rights in the expectation that they will be supported by the hospital
on behalf of its patients, as an integral part of the healing process. It is
recognized that a personal relationship between the physician and the
patient is essential for the provision of proper medical care. The traditional
physician–patient relationship takes on a new dimension when care is
rendered within an organizational structure. Legal precedent has established that the institution itself also has a responsibility to the patient.
It is in recognition of these factors that these rights are affirmed.

1. The patient has the right to considerate and respectful care.
2. The patient has the right to obtain from his physician complete current information concerning his diagnosis, treatment, and prognosis in
   terms the patient can be reasonably expected to understand. When it
   is not medically advisable to give such information to the patient, the
   information should be made available to an appropriate person in his
   behalf. He has the right to know, by name, the physician responsible
   for coordinating his care.
3. The patient has the right to receive from his physician information
   necessary to give informed consent prior to the start of any procedure
   and/or treatment. Except in emergencies, such information for informed consent should include but not necessarily be limited to the

specific procedure and/or treatment, the medically significant risks involved, and the probable duration of incapacitation. Where medically significant alternatives for care or treatment exist, or when the patient requests information concerning medical alternatives, the patient has the right to such information. The patient also has the right to know the name of the person responsible for the procedures and/or treatment.

4. The patient has the right to refuse treatment to the extent permitted by law and to be informed of the medical consequences of his action.

5. The patient has the right to every consideration of his privacy concerning his own medical care program. Case discussion, consultation examination, and treatment are confidential and should be conducted discretely. Those not directly involved in his care must have the permission of the patient to be present.

6. The patient has the right to expect that all communications and records pertaining to his care should be treated as confidential.

7. The patient has the right to expect that within its capacity a hospital must make reasonable response to the request of a patient for services. The hospital must provide evaluation, service, and/or referral as indicated by the urgency of the case. When medically permissible, a patient may be transferred to another facility only after he has received complete information and explanation concerning the needs for and alternatives to such a transfer. The institution to which the patient is to be transferred must first have accepted the patient for transfer.

8. The patient has the right to obtain information as to any relationship of his hospital to other health care and educational institutions insofar as his care is concerned. The patient has the right to obtain information as to the existence of any professional relationships among individuals, by name, who are treating him.

9. The patient has the right to be advised if the hospital proposes to engage in or perform human experimentation affecting his care or treatment. The patient has the right to refuse to participate in such research projects.

10. The patient has the right to expect reasonable continuity of care. He has the right to know in advance what appointment times and physicians are available and where. The patient has the right to expect that the hospital will provide a mechanism whereby he is informed by his physician or a delegate of the physician of the patient's continuing health care requirements following discharge.

11. The patient has the right to examine and receive an explanation of his bill regardless of source of payment.

12. The patient has the right to know what hospital rules and regulations apply to his conduct as a patient.

No catalog of rights can guarantee for the patient the kind of treatment he has a right to expect. A hospital has many functions to perform, including the prevention and treatment of disease, the education of both health professionals and patients, and the conduct of clinical research. All these activities must be conducted with an overriding concern for the patient, and, above all, the recognition of his dignity as a human being. Success in achieving this recognition assures success in the defense of the rights of the patient.

This formulation presents many problems. The rights it proclaims are not self-explanatory. It is unclear what they actually mean in specific cases. It is not clear whether exceptions exist and who shall arbitrate disputes. The document fails to distinguish between legally enforceable rights and other types of rights. This distinction can have great practical significance. Furthermore, the rights it proclaims are not self-enforcing. There are many reasons patients traditionally have been unable to assert or protect their rights. This document fails to assign responsibility for protecting the rights of patients to a person or to an office within the institution.

Nurses can play a role in reducing or eliminating these problems. First, serious thought and effort must be given to the development of a comprehensive and sound bill of rights for patients. In theory, such a document could play an important role in the health care process. It could be an expression of institutional and personal policy. It could clarify ambiguous areas of responsibility and liability. A well-written bill of rights could serve an educational role for both patients and providers. Such a document could also be a symbol of the acceptance of a new concept of the provider–patient relationship.

To be effective, such a document would have to distinguish between legally enforceable rights and other rights. It would have to represent a firm commitment to the concept of patient rights itself and avoid being no more than a consensus document developed through compromise and lacking real substance. Such a document would have to identify the mechanism for enforcing and protecting the rights of patients.

The development of an effective bill of patient rights should involve nurses as well as other health providers and patients. Nurses have too often been neglected or overlooked when the time for developing policy came. Nurses' insights need to be represented in this document.

It is my belief that the effectiveness of any bill of patient rights will depend in large part upon the effectiveness of the enforcement mechanism it contains. I believe that the most effective advocate for the patient would be an individual whose primary loyalty would be owed to the patient and not to the institution. I believe that a nurse should not be the formal patient advocate because of the many responsibilities she or he has as a care giver and as an employee of the institution. This does not in the least diminish her or his responsibility to identify and protect the rights of patients. It simply suggests a different focus for those concerns.

The process of developing such a document and such a mechanism will not be easy. It is a process that will take time, effort, and cooperation. But, it is a process with great potential for the cooperation of patient and provider. It is a process that nurses should welcome. However, in addition to the willingness and cooperative spirit which is needed, proper education and preparation for this leadership role is also necessary.

IV

Primary responsibility for preparing and encouraging the nurse to play an active leadership role in identifying and protecting the rights of patients rests with the schools of nursing. These schools must be committed to training nurses who possess both technical competence and sensitivity to their moral and legal obligations. There is no substitution for competence. Yet competence alone is not enough. Schools of nursing must be committed to the training of the whole nurse: as a competent health care provider, as a moral agent, as a legally responsible person. It is not difficult to see how the search for a more vital professional identity in nursing is related to the concept of patient rights. Schools of nursing should be committed to training health care providers for a vocation of service, shaped by the emerging provider–patient patterns of partnership rather than the traditional patterns of dominance. Schools of nursing should train their students for a leadership role in the identification and protection of patient rights. Out of such commitment can emerge a new sense of professional responsibility based on care for the patient as person. In the past, health care providers have been accused of two extreme reactions. The first, paternalism, was an error of excessive interference with the patient and the substitution of the provider as decision-maker. The second, indifference, was an error of insufficient concern for the patient. The concept of patient rights points the way to a middle ground between these extremes. The middle ground is compassion, an intention to serve without ignoring the patient as person. Such a concept could well become the distinctive characteristic of the "new" profession of nursing. During the past ten years, nurses have provided leadership in encouraging the discussion of critical issues in health care. I can only hope that they will once again avail themselves of this significant opportunity and demonstrate once again their courage and their dedication to a vocation of service to society.

Endnotes

1. E. Pellegrino, "Foreword" in *The New Health Professionals*, ed. A. Bliss and E. Cohen (Germantown, Maryland: Aspen Systems, 1977), p. xv.
2. S. Alsop, *Stay of Execution* (Philadelphia: J. B. Lippincott, 1973), pp. 10–11.

3. E. Cassell, *The Healer's Art* (Philadelphia: J. B. Lippincott, 1976), pp. 25–46.

4. B. Barber, "Compassion in Medicine: Toward New Definitions and New Institutions," *New England Journal of Medicine* 939, p. 295.

5. *See* L. Thomas, "The Health Care System" in *The Medusa and the Snail* (New York: Viking Press, 1979), pp. 45–50.

6. *See* J. Healey, "The Patient Viewpoint on Malpractice" in *Social Issues in Health Care*, ed. D. Self (Norfolk, Va.: Teagle and Little, 1977), p. 38.

7. Barber, "Compassion in Medicine."

8. In general, *see* G. Annas, *The Rights of Hospital Patients* (New York: Avon Press, 1975) and T. Beauchamp, and J. Childress *Principles of Biomedical Ethics* (New York: Oxford University Press, 1979).

9. *See* L. Besch, "Informed Consent: a Patient Right," *Nursing Outlook*, January 1979, pp. 32–35.

10. *See* N. Cantor, "A Patient's Decision to Decline Life-Saving Medical Treatment: Bodily Integrity versus the Preservation of Life," *Rutgers Law Review* 228 (1973), p. 26.

11. *See* U.S., Department of Health, Education, and Welfare, "Access to Medical Records," *Appendix, H.E.W. Secretary's Commission Report on Medical Malpractice,* (Washington, D.C.: U.S. Government Printing Office, 1973), pp. 186–213.

12. *See* A. Holder, *Medical Malpractice Law* (New York: John Wiley and Sons, 1978), p. 43.

13. *Ibid.,* p. 273.

14. *Ibid.,* p. 372.

Orgel points out that ethical dilemmas are the outcomes of the way we organize and conduct our social relations. He holds that we must investigate social conditions and reorganize social relations when possible in order to eliminate or reduce recurrent ethical dilemmas. Like Bertram Bandman, he maintains that the notion of moral autonomy as an absolute right perpetuates the conflicting claims of all parties in an ethical dilemma. He offers solutions to the problem of dealing with conflicting moral rights through focus on the process of making moral judgments and the process of establishing moral communities.

9

They Have No Right to Know: The Nurse and the Terminally Ill Patient

Gary S. Orgel

So-called ethical dilemmas can generally be shown to be products of the peculiar ways in which we have organized our social relations. That is, the choices we seem to be forced to make are often actually imposed upon us by the conditions antecedent to the choice that have themselves been created and perpetuated by the way we have constructed our social institutions. Solutions to these so-called dilemmas can be shown to consist not in a choice amongst the several alternative modes of action, but rather in the elimination of the preconditions for the necessity of making the choice.[1] That is to say that ethics, and particularly the ethics of health care, must not be a mere search for principles to which we allegedly can and must all conform. The world in which we live generates the ethical problems that it does precisely because we do not all hold the same world view or have common and uniform interests, and because most of us believe that this is the best way for a society to be organized. Thus, in choosing such a society it is simply folly to articulate any but the most fundamental principles in a way that supposes that we might all agree. The point is that conflicting views and interests are supported and legitimated in this society and it can only be in light of this recognition of conflict that ethics can proceed. Most ethical arguments proceed as if they can choose and legitimate the principles of one side of a debate, and by rational argument convince the opposing side to take an alternative position. But this is precisely what cannot, and in our society we agree need not, be done. Thus, those systems of ethics that merely accept the necessity of making a difficult choice without going further to investigate the antecedent and conflicting social conditions must necessarily fail to present themselves as practical and viable options, and thereby contribute to the maintenance of a conflict-ridden and unstable social structure.[2] In this sense any ethical perspective that is to be practical in the fullest sense of the word must address both the immediate need to make a choice and the questions concerning appropriate modes of reorganizing social relations so as to eliminate that need where possible in the future.[3]

I have been asked to address the problems raised by a situation in which a nurse has been ordered by his or her "superior" to refrain from informing a terminally ill patient that she or he is dying, under conditions in which the nurse genuinely believes that it would be in the patient's best interest to so inform him or her and where the nurse knows that no one else intends to undertake to tell the patient. I suggest that any solution to what has been called "the death dilemma" that merely rests on a notion of individual moral autonomy is inadequate. In the context of the nurse's problematic *vis a vis* her or his relations with physician and patient, it is wholly conceivable that the attempt to validate the moral autonomy of the nurse in terms of his or her rights may result in a violation of some right vested in the patient or physician. Similarly, if the nurse fulfills so-called duties to the patient or physician, his or her own sense of moral judgment may be infringed. In short, individual moral autonomy based either on notions of rights or duties merely perpetuates the conflicting claims of the parties.

While I suggest that every ethical system must claim to bestow some "good" upon the individual as such, it is not at all clear that this can be accomplished by mere individual action. This is particularly true where the special problems of the nurse are so enmeshed with a system of domination based on gender, and where the institutional organization in question has so developed its hierarchical structure that one profession amongst the many retains an inordinate amount of decision making authority.

We must distinguish here two concepts of authority. The first has as its essential feature a notion of power, whether it is socially legitimated power or the mere power created by the use of physical force. It is important to note that, while they are distinct, the two kinds of power share much, and indeed socially legitimated power may be the source of a great deal more dehumanizing activity than the power originating in force. In our society we have tended to ignore the possibility that authority that is legally validated may nevertheless be morally illegitimate. We have recognized that such authority can be abused, but that is not my point. What I am suggesting is hardly original and it is simply that legally or administratively valid authority is in no way necessarily connected to valid moral principles. The second kind of authority is that which is based on some notion of knowledge or skill. This may be either the mere possession of a collection of data as when we say "Jones is an authority on the anatomy of jelly fish," or it may be used to refer to a more holistic notion of knowledge as when we speak of a wise person. It is by no means accidental that we use the word *authority* in this second sense as a noun that refers to a person who *is* something, viz., an authority, by virtue of *having acquired* something else, viz., wisdom, while the first use of the word *authority* refers to something that is itself only possessed, as it were, from without. One sense of the word refers to the character of a person, while the other refers to a veneer painted on by other elements of the social structure. Now it may be the case that some socially legitimate authority is granted because one is recognized as an authority, but this need not be the case, and in any event this does not address the problem of the social obstacles to the acquisition of skills or wisdom. It also fails to address the problems created by the historical evolution of power relations between two groups which was not originally a function of evil intent or design, but which now is maintained precisely so that the predominance of one group can be enforced. We are thus faced with the possibility of a social institution which grants authority (*qua* power) by virtue of the recognition of wisdom and which simultaneously and systematically prevents certain individuals or groups from appropriating that skill, wisdom, or status.

The nurse, of course, is confronted with a multitude of persons in positions of superior authority, viz., other nurses with higher institutional status, hospital administrators, and doctors.[4] The question before us, framed as is usually the case in terms of an alleged right of the terminally ill patient to know the diagnosis of his or her condition, raises the question of the kind of authority the *patient* has over the nurse. In terms of authority the question can be phrased "Is the patient's right equivalent to having authority (*qua* power) or is the patient's authority derivative of the patient's right?"

I should like, therefore, to ask what it would mean to say that a patient has some absolute ethical right to receive information about a diagnosis of his or her impending death. I take it that to have such a right means that it would be wrong, regardless of the consequences, for everyone to withhold that information.[5] When a question is framed in terms of an absolute individual right there can be no question of considering consequences as mediating variables. If, for example, I have an absolute civil right to privacy it can make no difference that the majority or even all other people think it important to know and regulate what I do in my bedroom. A plebicite regarding such an absolute right renders it no right at all, for one essential aspect of having such a right is that a minority is protected from majority rule. It should be evident that on this strong definition of a right anything that is a right could not compete with anything else that is a right, and that the rights of individuals and groups could not compete with each other. Where rights compete, balancing right against right is the only way to settle claims. But balancing simply means that under certain conditions one has a right and under others one does not. In other words, once one engages in balancing rights one is no longer arguing that to have a right means that it would be wrong to prevent a person from actualizing that right. Under conditions of balancing one must argue that one can have a right and yet be interfered with in the actualization of that right. But this undermines the entire concept of a right by making it a wholly relative thing. Indeed the concept of right in our system of jurisprudence and in the language of contemporary ethics is precisely such a relative and shifting concept. Those who wish to opt for a strong definition of *right* will be hard pressed to find even one example of it anywhere in our social system. If, therefore, we were to assert that a patient had any absolute right to know her or his diagnosis, that would be perfectly consistent with the possibility that the patient might be harmed by such knowledge in so far as consequences cannot be counted as relevant when contending with an absolute right. Thus the health care professional might find him- or herself in the position of harming a patient in order to satisfy the claims of absolute right. If, on the other hand, we assert that such a right in the patient is relative and not absolute we would find ourselves pretending that as ethicists we could lay down some principle or set of principles that would actually help health care professions "properly balance" their rights *against* those of their patients. On the one hand, we would have to advise nurses to tell patients their diagnoses regardless of the consequences to the health of the patient, which is quite clearly absurd advice to give a health care professional of any sort. On the other hand, we would be forced to admit not only that there is a conflict between nurses and their patients but that an ethical response to that conflict consisted in a mere mediation of the antagonistic interests rather than their elimination. To take either position, the one implied by a theory of absolute right, the other implied by a theory of relative right, would fly in the face of the self-proclaimed roles of the nurse, viz., to advocate for one's patient and to do no harm to one's patient.

It is precisely for these reasons that I suggest that the language of rights and duties does not help the nurse, or indeed most of us, when we are confronted with an ethical problem. Rather we are aided much more by a discussion of the process of making moral judgments, and the process of establishing moral communities.[6] If we focus on the activities of moral reasoning and moral dialog we can, I think, find a way out of the box in which we find ourselves entrapped. This kind of perspective allows a consideration of, and includes, both perfectionist theories of the self and society and consequentialist theories. In fact, it cannot do without either, but it considers both in relation to one another. If I am to make myself as moral a person as I can be, but I must do this through social activity, then the results of that activity must have a bearing on the quality of the person I am becoming. Otherwise we should find ourselves in the peculiar situation of saying that one whose actions always resulted in harm to others could nevertheless be a moral person. Alternatively if the consequence of becoming a more morally sound person is not counted as one of the relevant consequences of my action, moral questions make no sense. For what would it mean to carry out the "right" action if that did not include, at least potentially, the effects that that action has or might have on all the relevant parties, and the moral agent is one of those parties. If I believe, as I do, that my own actions have an effect on me, then in considering proper moral conduct I must consider the effects of that action on my self. Thus, becoming a more morally sound person is necessarily entailed in a consideration of ethics. When we see that the objectives of moral reasoning and dialog simultaneously include the continued enhancement of my moral character and the well-being of others, attention is rightly focused on the moral development of a group and of each of its members. Moreover, in this view, the perfectionist and the consequentialist perspectives are unified and reconciled.

The question of honesty in the case of the nurse is intimately bound to the question of paternalism. The very necessity of asking whether we ought to tell a dying patient the true facts is itself a function of paternalism. One of the most destructive things about paternalism is that it is self-perpetuating. Those in the position of authority justify making decisions, and making decisions for others on the basis of superior knowledge, strength, intelligence, experience, or what have you. The point is, of course, that they are often correct about these facts, but only because either they have acted as a group, or the system of which they are a part is so ordered that inequality appears as a natural result. The facts those in power point to are not justifications, as they think they are, for their power, but rather symptoms of a system of domination.

We have produced a society of passive, indecisive patients. As an educator I must admit that that is precisely what we have done to our students as well. The infantilization of a variety of groups and classes in this society is characteristic of societies that have incorporated various modes of domination. We are forced to ask the kinds of questions about honesty now before us only when the passivity of the infantilized group begins to break down in certain ways. That is, we ask how much we should tell at some point in history when those "subordinate" to us begin to question our authority.

What we seek for a patient is not a mere abstract right to make decisions for and about him- or herself. Obviously the possession of facts is a necessary requisite to making an informed judgment, and for this reason we have treated the question of what to tell the dying patient as essentially one of facts. Making an informed judgment, however, presupposes the ability and willingness to make judgments. But this is precisely the problem. Making decisions well is a function of having practiced making decisions, and this is true for the nurse as well as the patient. Making decisions is often treated as essentially a process that goes on "in the head" of a particular individual. No doubt, all decisions are products of the thought processes of discrete individuals. But the most rational decisions are those that are a product of the examination of the multitude of facets of the problem. In other words, rationality depends on a union and reconciliation of diverse values and perspectives. While much of this may be achievable by one person, Plato was quite right in recognizing that only through dialog, examining and counter-examining, questioning and answering is a thorough working through of a problem possible. Of course in moral discourse we are not concerned merely with rationality. In some cases it may be imprudent not to consult others but it would not necessarily be unethical. With respect, however, to situations involving a patient, action on his or her behalf requires a consideration of his or her *actual* perspective, and this involves moral dialog. The final decision must, therefore, emerge from this dialog and be consistent with the perspectives of the various parties. Our problems today are grounded to a large extent in the fact that "clinical conferences" have not in the past included nurses or patients, while such dialogs are common to the practice of doctors. Those who have made decisions in the past have always engaged in dialog amongst themselves to determine what is "best" for the patient. We are now aiming at including more people in precisely those dialogs already in process. The questions are whether being a nurse or a patient entails the expectation that one will be included in decision making and whether doctors are willing to fully admit nurses and patients into the decision making process.

For the nurse, the problem is one of concentrating on the actualization of the most extensive decision making ability of a particular patient given all relevant conditions. This may, and at some point must, include facts, but sharing facts is only part of a larger scheme, and taken by itself may be either a helpful or destructive act. It may be caring or it may be harmful. It may be respectful or it may be degrading. The issue upon which the nurse must continually focus is the development of the patient's ability to make actual decisions about his or her life, and indeed given the amount of time the nurse spends with patients, he or she is eminently qualified to fulfill this role.

The particular characteristics of the patient as regards her or his ability or need to hear or understand various issues can only be known by those who spend sufficient time with the patient. Only they can have insight into a patient's uniqueness. The issue is one of responding to the existential demands of a given situation, guided by the principle that optimally every patient should be put in an emotional and psychological condition that allows her or him to participate fully in the decisions that affect her or his life and death. In many cases the emotional or psychological condition of the patient when she or he is presented to the hospital staff will be such that the task will never be fulfilled. But this is still the goal and guiding principle and must not be subordinated to shallow rules that demand that all mere facts be revealed regardless of consequences.

Now all of this presupposes a condition that I described before, that is, the condition of patient passivity and indecisiveness, patient fear and denial. It is hardly a laudable situation but it is the one we have. The whole idea is not to remain at this impoverished level where physicians and nurses are forced to squabble with each other about the appropriate way to parent their children! I have supposed, furthermore, that there was a disagreement between nurse and physician about whether to tell a patient that she or he was dying, and the condition for the possibility for such disagreement must be either a disagreement about the facts regarding the state of the patient, or some moral conflict as to precisely what the actual goal ought to be. If they tell the truth they may do harm to the patient. If they fail to tell all the facts they believe they are undermining a patient's ability to participate in that decision making which affects her or his life. Both positions are correct, and the choice is not dependent on discovering which position is more correct. Rather, it is dependent on walking the narrow ridge that demands both that you do no harm and that self-determination is always particular to an individual. Self-determination is not just any freedom to make any decision. It is the specific capacity to make specific decisions. The nurse, precisely because of his or her intimate connections with the particular and unique characteristics of a patient, must be called upon to make judgments based on perceptions of the patient's capacities and must encourage the development of those capacities.

At the beginning of this paper I asserted that so-called ethical dilemmas can generally be shown to be products of the ways in which we have organized our social structure. I then proceeded to emphasize the nature of the authority relations—relations based on power and status that govern the institutional life of doctors and nurses. Now I should like to point to the fact that nurses have already begun the struggle for equal authority in the decision making process. How are these three points related in regard to ethical problems that health care professionals face? We would all agree, I believe, that we could not hold a person morally blameworthy for an action undertaken as a result of coercion or duress. That is, while if we are to engage in ethical dialog at all we must *assume* that the parties to the discussion are free moral agents, it is nevertheless conceivable that in certain situations conditions of constraint operate that affect the nature of the so-called freedom of the moral agent. In this paper I am addressing people who are confronted with the necessity of making decisions within the confines of an institutional framework. Now the nation in which we live, with its unique socioeconomic conditions, the institutions in which we work or play, the homes in which we live, all establish *in the first instance* the limits within which we make our decisions. Most are presented to us as "facts" of the social world at our birth. Some, on the other hand, we create ourselves. If, for example, I am born into a monogamous family unit with two older siblings, the limits within which I must make decisions are different from, say, those for one born of a polygamous union with fifteen older children. "Limit" is, oddly enough, a way to denote context. That is, things thought of as the "outer" reaches of a situation (i.e., its limits) are indicative of the internal structure of that situation. Thus, *limit* and *context* are reciprocal terms. Every decision we are called upon to make is a decision to be made within a *definite* set of limits, and thus in a *definite* context. If this is true then several choices follow: (1) we are all free moral agents irrespective of context and limits, and we are thus wholly accountable for all our moral decisions, or (2) the existence of limits and contexts in which we must make decisions is *equivalent* to the existence of constraints upon us and, therefore, no one is rightly held accountable for so-called moral decisions because no one can act in a way that is free of coercion, or (3) that we make decisions in definite contexts with definite limits is itself morally neutral, and is in fact the necessary requisite to making decisions and moral decisions at all. But, and this is crucial for us, *certain* contexts, and *certain* limits may be coercive or constraining, and thus the moral accountability of persons acting under such constraints is called into question. Now I hope that it is evident to my readers that I am arguing for this third alternative. That is, all moral judgments are social judgments and, therefore, contextual judgments. To eliminate the context or limits of a situation from a consideration of the nature of a judgment is precisely to eliminate the conditions for the possibility of making a judgment at all. But we are not merely speaking of contextual judgments in general. What we seek are judgments that are right and good. That is, the very fact that anyone asks a question of him- or herself in regard to *possible* future action is itself indicative of the fact that not only are we as humans forced to choose our future course of action, but we always ask questions about these courses of action in terms of definite values, principles, or ideals. In fact, to see "x" and "y" as possible courses of future action implies that in order to choose "x," "y," "x and y," "not-x," "not-y," or "not-x and not-y" I must have a value hierarchy, even if it is unconscious or arbitrary, by which to choose. But then that is precisely why every single judgment we make both is contextual and has ethical implications (no matter how narrow they may be). So, to make any sense at all about making judgments about possible courses of action, we need to have reference both to a definite context and to a set of values. In the absence of one or the other we would have the absurd situation of either having precisely nothing about which to deliberate (no context) or no knowledge that a choice was involved (things would not be regarded as possibilities) in which case no judgment would be required.

Now, if it is the case that social context and limits are not equivalent to constraints, then it follows that it is not the case that making ethical judgments in a particular institutional context is itself problematic. Where, however, the limits of decision making are grounded in relations of power (i.e., authority) it is quite a different matter. Relations based on power are relations that inhibit the ability of the subordinate group to make judgments, as well as its ability to act. That is, power affects both the thought processes and the social action of the subordinate group. We are taught to "respect" those in power. It thus becomes a problem for nurses whether they ought to value the doctors' orders because they are the doctors', or value them because they are the right orders. But we know that whenever someone carries out "someone else's" orders, the act implies that *all things considered* this is believed to be the right thing to do by the person carrying out the orders. That is, either the person has decided that it is more important to "follow orders" than to evaluate the substantive legitimacy of those orders, or he or she finds the substance of the orders to be in accord with his or her own sense of that which is right. But history demands that we admit that, where the substance of those orders is unethical, "I was just following orders" is not an answer to a charge of immoral conduct. But we are a self-contradictory society! We want a respect for those in power, and we also want to hold subordinates morally responsible for their own actions. We teach both of these values in the military, in religious institutions, in schools, and with respect to the relations we have to the government in general. We cannot have it both ways. Power relations are relations of constraint and place subordinate groups under duress. These subordinate groups, of which nurses are one, cannot make ethical judgments just insofar as they are "under orders" to act in a particular way, and real social forces of an administrative, legal, or economic sort operate to coerce nurses into acting in accordance with orders from superiors. But if power relations are relations of constraint, then all forms of these relations are themselves ethically illegitimate. To constrain someone is to render that person something less than human, for to be human necessarily entails the ability to socially engage oneself in discourse aimed at discovering the right action to take in the future. Furthermore, this ability is rendered barren and impotent if one does not *know* at the onset that one's values and analyses count as much as the values and analyses of anyone else engaged in the dialog.

Thus the abolition of power relations, relations whose extreme is the master-slave relationship, is a precondition for the possibility of not merely the existence of ethical individuals, but an ethical society! An institution in which people are forced to act under orders is an unethical institution as such, and no one in the institution can claim to be free of the taint of illegitimacy, even if the substance of the orders is itself "legitimate." The form has betrayed the content!

Who then is to abolish these power relations, these relations of constraint? Can it be the ones in power? This would produce the absurd situation of the benificent dictator "granting" democracy to his or her people. A people must be ready for democracy, and the concrete proof comes to light when they demand responsibility for their own actions. The abolition of constraint cannot come from the top, for this, once again only appears to be substantively legitimate. It appears to eliminate relations of constraint. But it does so precisely in the form of those relations that it claims to abolish. Those in authority *order* its abolition! What is missing is the ethical consciousness of the subordinate group which proclaims "we demand to be fully responsible for what we choose to do." But it is just this consciousness that has begun to emerge amongst nurses. This consciousness, being the precondition for the possibility of ethical action is the first indication to us all that nurses are becoming morally responsible people. Both the Nazi doctor at Nuremberg and the contemporary nurse who follows a doctor's orders are tragic characters. They are tragic just because they are indeed doing just what the society says they ought to be doing, viz., following orders, and at the same time failing to fulfill their responsibilities to their patients, the other thing society demands of them. The two social values are in direct opposition to each other, and thus nurses are in a lose-lose situation, damned if they do and damned if they don't.

But this then brings us back to the political, legal, and ethical question of the authority that the nurse's judgment should have when it conflicts with that of the physician either as regards information to be imparted to a patient or the treatment that is appropriate for a patient. As a matter of institutional authority the issue is easily resolved if one makes the will of the patient controlling and not merely contributory. Whoever can get the patient to agree with her or him wins the authority struggle. The problem with this model is precisely that it is a conflictual model. It sounds precisely like something that should be settled by an administrative body or a court of law. In fact, it smacks of a child custody hearing in which the mother and father battle over the child, and the battle itself, regardless of the outcome, raises the specter of endangering the welfare, happiness, and security of the child. Indeed this is precisely the way in which problems like this are being settled in some parts of the country, and decisions have not been particularly favorable to the moral integrity or authority of the nurse. The point is precisely that so long as these situations arise as conflictual *per se* and not as mere disagreements amongst equals who have common goals and share common background beliefs they cannot but be settled by courts, and those settlements will legitimate, at least for the forseeable future, the current system with its hierarchical structure. Internal conflict based on professional and gender domination is anathema to the welfare of the patient. Now, I say that conflict is anathema to the welfare of the patient, for indeed the patient fared reasonably well, indeed in some senses even fared better where gender and professional domination was an accepted mode of institutional and social organization. One obvious response to this problem, therefore, is to eliminate the conflict by supressing rebellious women and nurses. It may at first glance appear to be a silly suggestion, but history teaches us that it is inevitably the first response of those whose power is threatened, and that of the legal system that stands behind them. But it is only the first response. Even today there are already sensitive and enlightened doctors prepared to meet nurses as equals and who are willing to dispense with the services of judge and jury in the quest for solutions to moral problems.

The question of equality is a serious question for several reasons. First, there is no clear social consensus on what the word means. Second, the historical hegemony of the male and of the doctor in medical education, practice, and research lends credence to the claim that with respect to knowledge and skill physicians are superior to nurses and, therefore, should enjoy greater authority. Third, while it is possible that the preceeding claim is true, but not at all clear that it is true, doctors and nurses need each other. They are, by virtue of the historical evolution of the professions, interdependent parts of a greater whole. The physician cannot act without cooperative nurses and indeed for some very specific reasons cannot in many cases even make appropriate clinical judgments without the cooperation and advice of nurses.

The meaning of equality is something that history and continued moral dialog will need to work out. As to the implications for equality in the sense of medical knowledge and skill, the resolution to this problem will be partly, but only partly, settled by the struggle of nurses and nursing schools to demonstrate that the quality of their education meets and will continue to meet the rigorous demands of medical science. But equality should not be confused with sameness. Nurses do not have to prove that they are really a subspecialty of the category "physician" in order to qualify as the equal of physicians. Indeed, what we are moving toward, and what is heralded by the current self-assertiveness of the nursing profession, is a recognition that nurses, physicians, and others must be unified under a category common to all, whose characteristics are determined by the various professions included under it or fighting to be included under it. Short of this neither nurses nor physicians can consistently be committed to the welfare of their patients, for their own internal conflict undermines that welfare.

Once a group demands to be treated as an equal that movement toward equality cannot be halted short of actual suppression. The growing complexity of medical institutions, the reliance of these institutions on great numbers of nurses, and the increasing refinement of nursing education amongst other things have all made the modern physician acutely aware of the significance of the nurse. This reliance on the nurse is both the ground upon which to build the empirical struggle for equal authority and the philosophical basis for asserting that if the physician is unable to successfully define the parameters of his or her functions without reference to the nurse, and if the nurse is cognizant of this dependence and demands as a consequence that she or he be responsible for those decisions made as a function of this dependence, then the nurse must already be an equal collaborator of the physician in some sense.[7]

Several things follow from this. First, disagreement on clinical and moral matters is not itself problematic amongst persons of equal authority. It is, or can be, a source of development and learning. When equals disagree, and to the extent that they respect and know each other as equals, they agree on ground rules for playing the game in the event of disagreement. There are no rules for the philosopher to offer for how disagreements should be settled. This must be left to the distinct persons and groups engaged in moral dialog. The only rule that can be offered refers to the equality of the participants and this must ultimately be recognized both by nurses and physicians. To fail to recognize it is necessarily to undermine patient care, and that would involve nurses and physicians in a palpable self-contradiction. Nurses who adopt the passive, indecisive role fail to recognize that in many cases only they have access to special information requisite to a proper clinical judgment, and that only they can provide many types of essential patient care and can do so only on their own initiative.[8] They also run the risk of contributing to medical error where, for example, they dutifully follow directions that in their best clinical judgment are wrong and result in harm to the patient. Physicians who fail to recognize nurses as equals fail to see the emerging realities of the collapse of traditionally male-dominated paternalistic systems. Moreover, they fail to acknowledge their reliance on the skill and wisdom of nurses in making clinical judgments. Physicians who stubbornly hold on to the reins of power encourage and enhance a condition of conflict in the institutions in which they are allegedly caring for their patients.[9]

It is in the ultimate interest of patients therefore, that nurses, acting as a group and individually, continually struggle to insist upon playing an equal role in making decisions. We must pay a price for past offenses. The transition from oppression to equal authority will not be a completely smooth one, and each group will be hurt somewhat in the ensuing struggle. Great care must be taken to ensure a minimum of harm to the patients, particularly to their sense of security and willingness to trust the health care professionals with whom they must work. Individual nurses will be called upon to exhibit moral courage and refuse to follow orders where those orders immediately conflict with their best moral or clinical judgment, and where they have exhausted all dialectical channels by which to come to some agreement with alleged superiors. Ultimately every health care professional must be convinced that the action he or she is about to take is clinically and morally justified. If they are not so convinced what are the grounds upon which they carry out that act? The nurse who is courageous in this regard must not be asked to stand alone.[10] She or he must be able to rely on the group of nurses with whom she or he works and even on state and national groups for moral support. This means that nursing groups must be prepared to take action to protect themselves, their interests, and the interests of their patients. What we are seeking is the greatest freedom possible with the least amount of institutional disruption necessary. But we cannot expect that there will be no institutional disruption. We can only hope that all parties will realize that their commitments to patients demand that as many dialectical channels as possible be opened and kept open, and that institutional struggles be settled by the main participants in the struggle, and not by third-party mediators like courts of law. For better or for worse, the analogies to the family that I have used in this paper break down in the final analysis because there can be no divorce between nurse and physician.

Endnotes

1. One may be tempted to suggest that what is being described here is political and not ethical action. The two are, however, inextricably tied, and particularly for nurses and other health care professionals. Because their individual action proceeds, generally and for the most part, within the context of institutions, the analysis must not be presented as if it is sufficient to consider mere individual actors and actresses. Institutional designs establish the parameters of action and one must address both the nature of actions possible within *given* parameters and the legitimacy of those parameters themselves.

2. *See,* for example, B. I. Chazan, "The Moral Situation" in *Moral Education,* ed. J. F. Soltis and B. I. Chazan (New York: Teachers College Press, 1973), pp. 39–49.
3. Note that I do not eschew the real need to make choices nor do I suggest that these decisions are in any way ethically trivial. What I do suggest is that unless they are tied to a broader institutional ethic the choices made will be both shortsighted and impotent.
4. Whether we use a Weberian or Bernardian scheme of authority structures, it is in the interface of authority, rationality, and dialog in the decision making process that we find the limits of the nurses' clinical and moral problems set. *See* T. K. Hopkins, "Bureaucratic Authority: The Convergence of Weber and Bernard" in *Complex Organizations: A Sociological Reader,* ed. A. Etzioni, (New York: Holt, Rinehart and Winston, 1962).
5. *See,* for example, R. Dworkin, *Taking Rights Seriously,* (Cambridge, Mass.: Harvard University Press, 1977).
6. *See* M. Buber, "The Education of Character" in *Between Man and Man,* (New York: Macmillan Press, 1972).
7. The so-called ritualistic adherence to established policy that appears to be associated with nursing practice is contrasted in an enlightening manner to questions of innovative acting in R. L. Coser, "Authority and Decision Making in a Hospital: A Comparative Analysis," in *Readings on Modern Organization,* ed. A. E. Etzioni (Englewood Cliffs, N.J.: Prentice-Hall, 1969).
8. *See* I. G. Mauksch, "The Paradox of Risk Takers," *AORN Journal* 25 (1977), pp. 1289ff. in which a profile of the nurse is offered from studies done through 1962. The nurses' characteristics include: great need for submissiveness, order, blame avoidance, and a low need for risk taking.
9. In Milgram's excellent work *Obedience to Authority* (New York: Harper and Row, 1974), the author indicated precisely how the social context can operate to command obedience to even the most morally offensive orders. It is encouraging to note that if we assume that doctor's orders may sometimes be morally misguided but are unlikely to be heinous in character, it is nevertheless the case that these mildly offensive orders have stirred the minds and passions of nurses.
10. *See* L. Y. Kelly, "The Patient's Right to Know," *Nursing Outlook* 24 (1976), pp. 26–32 for a characterization of some of the problems such a "courageous" nurse might face.

Selected Bibliography

Annas, George J. "Rights of the Terminally Ill Patient." *Journal of Nursing Administration* 4 (1974): 40–44.
Aronson, G. J. "Treatment of the Dying Person," in *The Meaning of Death,* (New York: McGraw-Hill, 1959), pp. 251–58.

Browning, Mary H., and Lewis, Edith P. comps. *Nursing and the Cancer Patient.* New York, American Journal of Nursing, 1973.

Bunch, Barbra, and Zahra, Donna. "Dealing with Death—the Unlearned Role." *American Journal of Nursing* 76 (1976).

Cassell, Eric. "Death and the Physician." *Commentary*, June 1969, pp. 73–79.

Caughill, Rita E., ed. *The Dying Patient: A Supportive Approach.* Boston: Little, Brown, 1976.

Clinical Care Committee of the Massachusetts General Hospital. "Optimum Care for the Hopelessly Ill Patients." *New England Journal of Medicine* 295 (1976): 362–364.

Downie, P. A. "Symposium: Care of the Dying; A Personal Commentary on the Care of the Dying on the North American Continent." *Nursing Mirror* 139 (1974): 68–70.

Montange, Charles H. "Informed Consent and the Dying Patient." *Yale Law Journal* 83 (July 1974): 1632–74.

Pine, Vanderlyn R. "Institutionalized Communication About Dying and Death." *Journal of Thanatology* 3 (1975): 1–12.

In discussing the patient's right to reject treatment, Aroskar points out the frequent conflict between the patient's individualism and self-determination as an ultimate value and the interests of community and those caring for the patient. She rejects the extreme position of self-determination as the guiding ethic and, like Bertram Bandman and Orgel, she recommends that we consider the individual patient in the context of a community that involves the patient as well as those affected by the decision.

10

A Nursing Perspective on the Right of the Patient to Reject Treatment

Mila Aroskar

Who should make what choices, and where, in the process of making decisions around the suffering individual who refuses a specific treatment or who begs the nurse to be allowed to die? Does an individual have a "right" to make any choices whatsoever, or are there some limits to the choices? If there are limits, what is the basis of these limits? These are key questions for nurses, patients, and others who are participants in ethical dilemmas characterized by conflict and equally unattractive alternatives for action. In this paper, the suffering individual is referred to as a patient, although it is recognized that in some settings the preferred label is "client."

Making decisions is often viewed as a linear process. However, in the complexity of living, dying, loving, working, and interrelating, decisions more often seem to be reflective of a mosaic of past choices, both rational and non-rational. All these choices impinge on a given situation at a given point in time in the processes of being born, living, and dying. In these situations, critical decisions must often be made with, or for, an individual by others in given social roles. These others may be health professionals or family members involved with the individual patient in making choices related to acceptance or rejection of treatment. At times, the courts or hospital ethics committees may also make decisions around such issues.

Any one choice by an individual to accept or reject a specific treatment may or may not lead to death with varying degrees of probability. This uncertainty of outcomes makes talking about a "right" to choose in this area terribly ambiguous for all those involved. To whom in a hospital or community does one present the claim of such a "right?" Who, if anyone, has the obligation or duty to assure such a "right?" No one can predict with certainty whether a choice to reject a specific treatment, such as chemotherapy, will cause death. One is not choosing death or life *per se,* but whether or not to participate in a specific treatment or procedure which may or may not alter the time of one's own death, but which may well alter the quality of one's living. In making choices of this nature, one does have statistical probabilities as part of the input, but it is significant to all involved that no one can predict the outcome for any specific individual.

Talk about making decisions related to ethical dilemmas in certain patient care settings is generally talk about decisions that involve a critical aspect in relation to time constraints. Physician, nurse, and patient are enmeshed in situations where decisions must be made for a particular action or inaction in a given time frame. Each alternative has consequences which cannot be predicted totally by anyone. The decision making process, as mentioned earlier, involves not just one major decision but several intermediate decisions with many contingencies, such as which physician or emergency room one initially chooses to visit for diagnosis and treatment, whose advice one uses in making this decision, and when one seeks to enter the health care delivery system, along the way.

Whatever setting of care, treatment, and decision making one is talking about, whether home, hospital, physician's office, or neighborhood health center, the nurse or nursing is often the interface between the patient, physician, and family. Examples of this interface or nurse-in-the-middle position, are relaying or reinforcing information from the physician or other health workers, helping the patient negotiate the system, carrying out physician-ordered treatments, and initiating nursing care and comfort measures to promote an environment more supportive of the patients' own healing powers and wishes.

In this position of interface with dying persons, the nurse is in a unique position as demonstrated in the findings of a research project conducted at two Seattle hospitals where nurses' attitudes toward euthanasia and dying were studied. Findings included the following: (1) nurses more frequently hear patient requests for positive or direct euthanasia than physicians do, and (2) nurses are more comfortable working with physicians who let patients die than physicians who pursue vigorous treatment in a situation that can only be identified at a given moment in time as hopeless.[1] These study findings are reflective of the position of the individual nurse and nursing as a service vis-a-vis patients. They may also reflect personal and professional feelings and values related to patient rights to self-determination and self-responsibility, obedience of the nurse, use of coercion to achieve certain ends, use of "heroic" measures, and the value which says that death may not be the worst thing that can happen to an individual given certain circumstances.

Self-Determination as Ultimate Value

Can the nurse and physician, then, be viewed as individual moral agents free to make decisions about patient care where the patient's self-determination is the ultimate value? If self-determination is accepted by everyone as a basic value, a moral principle, or perhaps an absolute "right," health professionals and families could not question a "right" to accept or reject treatment. On this extreme position, the "right" of the patient to exercise self-determination is a given and overrides any other considerations, such as consequences for others of a given decision. Obviously, then, the patient can choose to accept or reject treatment generally or specific treatments following a completely individualistic ethic.

Before one accepts this as an acceptable position or principle, even though individualism is a strong value in our society, one should give due consideration to other requirements suggested by Rawls for principles of right. These requirements include that principles should: (1) be general in terms of reasonableness and of equal advantage to all, (2) be universal in their application in terms of the consequences if everyone adheres to them, (3) be known to all, (4) order conflicting claims, and (5) act as a final court of appeal, overriding existing laws and customs.[2] These considerations rule out an egoistic position in which the nurse does what is most comfortable for him or her without considering the possibility of a moral principle as a guide to action or thinking about the consequences of a given decision for the patient and others affected by the decision.

Are we as individuals or a society willing to accept self-determination as an ultimate value? If we answer in the affirmative, then the next question is for whom should this be the ultimate value when decision makers conflict in any given situation? Are we willing to accept that individuals may then make tragic choices for themselves? How can this value be universalized to all involved in a given situation and what are the consequences if everyone adheres to self-determination as an ultimate value? What are the consequences for the larger community and for society if self-determination is treated as the final court of appeal by individuals who wish to reject specific treatments? This position could and does often conflict with the traditional medical ethic which says that everything should be done to preserve the life of the individual. This medical ethic represents a paternalistic stance, which could make the health professional's values the overriding consideration in any given patient care situation—not a generally desirable situation.

Should we also not view others and ourselves as interconnected members of a system or a community of particular interests and concerns of caring? The value of community is often lost in the pursuit of individualism in the sense that the interests of others who care about the suffering individual and society are also involved in decisions made by and about individuals who comprise a given community. Other individuals, such as family members, also suffer the consequences of decisions to accept or reject a treatment such as renal dialysis.

To make self-determination the ultimate criterion for making decisions seems to point in the direction of a lonely, isolated collection of individuals that negates and denies the underlying interdependence and connectedness of the individuals, in this case, the physician, nurse, patients, and families, within a social system and a community. Rollo May, in his book *Power and Innocence,* claims that we are indeed searching for community because we have lost the sense of community that involves understanding and mutual valuing by members of a given community. The notion of a community may indicate a geographic or political entity, or perhaps a common interest group. It is within the relationships of a human community that the rights of individuals emerge.

If an individual chooses not to recognize a sense of community in making decisions related to life and death, then perhaps this individual has an obligation not to present him- or herself at an institution such as a hospital, since, under current circumstances, going to a hospital generally means making health professionals the primary decision makers. This is often a reality to be faced in spite of posted declarations of patient rights and employment of patient advocates in some hospitals. Hospitals as social institutions are expected to express a sense of connectedness with and responsibility for the sick and suffering in the community. I am thinking here specifically of the individual who would reject particular treatments of self without consideration of consequences to others. Such an individual might feel that life is no longer worth living, given particular circumstances. Such situations range from an individual who has just been given a diagnosis of cancer, to an elderly person receiving life-saving treatment, to a person in uncontrollable pain. A key question for all involved is whether life is being maintained or suffering is being prolonged. This is not always an easy differentiation to make in light of many physical, psychological, emotional, and cultural unknowns.

Both individuals and professions seem to be caught in the tension between an ethic of extreme individualism and freedom of self-determination and an ethic of community connectedness and cooperation in talking about rights. In an ethic emphasizing individualism, feedback within the individual person, patient or professional, takes priority, by means of a selective listening process, over feedback from others. The patient ignores feedback from others who are essentially healthy and separate from him- or herself, for example, the terminally ill, lucid patient who seeks to die versus the family members, nurses, physicians who want the individual to live for a variety of reasons expressive of certain personal, professional, or institutional values. The patient's attempt to ignore feedback from others by asserting extreme individualism is carried on at a price to all concerned in the decision making process, where individual decisions affect others in the system directly or indirectly, for example, where the patient is the mother of a young family, a loved child, a corporate executive. These individuals are all decision makers in a complex set of interpersonal relationships where everyone involved will experience the social, psychological, or financial consequences of a given decision.

Terminally ill or dying patients are also in an ambiguous situation related to the sick role and the expectations for this role, such as seeking appropriate help and cooperating with that help in order to return to one's accustomed social roles. Do physicians and nurses have different duties and obligations to the sick person who does not or cannot fulfill these role expectations? Can they opt out of caring for these persons who cannot be cured and who also refuse available treatment(s)? An affirmative answer to this question has serious implications for many individuals with chronic illnesses who do not follow treatment regimens for a variety of known and unknown reasons. The nurse is in a key position in a community or institutional network where he or she gets feedback and input from patients, physicians, family members, and administrators in many health care settings as noted in the previously cited research.

Are nurses, too, struggling to develop a professional ethic of individualism and autonomy for themselves and patients which negates an ethic of community responsibility and connectedness? If one accepts the right to self-determination for all involved in a patient–health worker relationship as a significant value in decision making, then would not anarchy and chaos prevail in health and medical care institutions? The team concept in health care is negated by the health worker's insistence on an individualistic ethic for the health professional. Or, should one indeed argue for acceptance of what Veatch, a philosopher, calls an "engineering model" of relationships where the patient's wishes (rights) prevail?[3] Under this model, nurses and physicians simply do what the patient wants them to do as technicians and applied scientists. Their values are not taken into consideration in the decision making process and they simply service the patient's wishes. This kind of relation has significant implications for the personal and professional integrity of nurses and physicians and also makes certain assumptions about the patient's knowledge and expertise in matters of health and illness. Acceptance of this model for decision making ignores those patients at the other end of the continuum who wish the professional to make all important decisions related to their care and treatment.

Community Alternatives

In thinking and talking about social, system, and institutional rearrangements to meet individual patients' needs and prevent some critical patient care dilemmas, perhaps we should consider whether or not we want institutions such as hospitals where patients and their families can assume that everything will be done to maintain and preserve life, to cure if at all possible. What if communities chose to support at least two types of institutions, one adhering to the traditional medical ethic and one where the underlying ethic was that of preserving a certain quality of life? The consequences in terms of who received certain resources and who did not receive these resources could be alarming. Some of these consequences have occurred in relation to allocation of resources for renal dialysis in the past. Or communities might identify needs for institutions differentiated according to a primary focus on curing and a primary focus on caring when cure is not possible.

Physicians and nurses dedicated to an ethic of preserving life may not be the most appropriate decision makers or care takers in relation to patients identified as terminally ill and dying. *Caring for and being with rather than curing* become the predominant focus of decisions and activity in these situations according to the theologian, Paul Ramsey, who has developed an ethics of caring for the dying in his book, *The Patient as Person. Caring for* the individual is indeed an obligation which raises questions as to how health professionals learn to accept or fulfill this kind of obligation which is expressive of particular values somewhat different from those generally underlying the behaviors of health professionals related to curing, such as valuing "being with" an individual in addition to "doing for" an individual relative to his or her physical/psychological condition. In an action-oriented society that values efficiency, the value of simply "being with" someone is not easy to adopt and express.

Ramsey points out that those who may get well require particular kinds of assistance, whereas those who are dying require different responses from health professionals. He says that the claims of the "suffering-dying" upon the human community are "quite different" from the claims of those who will still live though suffering or those who are incurably ill but not dying yet.[4] In considering care for the dying, it is imperative that nurses think about the structural changes needed in institutions on patient care units and the profound changes required in professional values and behaviors to solve what has been identified as the chief problem of the dying, how not to die alone.[5] This may become even more critical for the dying person who directly challenges the traditional medical ethic and rejects treatment. Can one automatically assume that this individual will receive needed care on a busy patient care unit? Every health professional may not be able to participate effectively in care for the dying whether in the hospital or at home if this is too threatening to values held by an individual nurse or physician. Acknowledgment of this possibility is an argument against the engineering model mentioned previously, which does not take into account a nurse's own values in a nurse–patient relationship.

The Joseph Saikewicz decision by the Supreme Court in Massachusetts seems at least to recognize the question whether physicians and other health professionals are the appropriate decision makers in relation to discontinuing use of life-sustaining mechanisms or witholding of treatment that is life prolonging but not curative. Courts were made the decision makers in the Saikewicz decision, whereas in the Quinlan decision ethics committees were required to have input into these decisions. These decisions still do not resolve the question definitively as to who should most appropriately make these decisions. Legal decisions do not necessarily meet the requirements of moral decision making.

Hospices provide an example of an institutional arrangement predicated on a primary orientation and value of *care* rather than the acute care hospital setting where the primary value is *cure*. Maybe the caring relationship can be designed into organizations having this specific purpose. This is not to minimize the need for an "underlying consensual caring" in all of a community's institutions. One idea, expressed by Mayeroff in his book *On Caring* suggests that:

> To care for another person, I must be able to understand him and his world as if I were inside it. I must be able to see, as it were, with his eyes what his world is like to him and how he sees himself. Instead of merely looking at him in a detached way from outside, as if he were a specimen, I must be able to be with him in his world, "going" into his world in order to sense from "inside" what life is like for him, what he is striving to be, and what he requires to grow.[6]

This notion of caring has profound implications for nurses and others involved with dying individuals. What are the personal costs or benefits to individuals who choose to work in such settings? Can society afford such options? On the other hand, can we afford not to have these options available for those with particular needs?

Already existing caring must be identified and reinforced as an individual, institutional, and community-wide value.[7] Alternatives of the sort mentioned previously could provide patients and families with choices where the issue is not acceptance or rejection of treatment *per se,* but a choice for a particular type of support system while living. Communities, in the larger sense of community, can provide options more responsive to patient need rather than seek to make one institution such as the hospital serve all patient needs on the living-dying continuum. A decision to provide options seems to recognize in a more sensitive and humane way that both professionals and patients have different needs and values.

Respect for the Individual as a Value

In rejecting an extreme position on self-determination as an ultimate value in talking about the patient's "right" to reject treatment, since in reality the "right" to *accept* treatment has not been challenged, the value of respect for the individual might be posited as an alternative notion. Nurses at the interface between physicians and patients, for example, are in a unique position to assure that this value is expressed in the decision making process, although this does not mean that it will be easy to follow through on the assurance. Respect for individuals requires that each individual be treated in consideration of his or her uniqueness, as equal to every other, and that special justification is required for interference with an individual's purposes, privacy, or behavior.[8]

The concept of respect for the individual requires that a minimum consideration in decision making affecting the suffering individual is that the individual's own desires be considered in any decisions that affect his or her current or future welfare. This rules out a paternalistic stance in decision making where health professionals make decisions with no consideration of the patient's own values and wishes.

If respect for the individual were made a guiding ethical principle for the nurse (nursing)–patient relationship, it could affect both individual interactions on patient-care units and nursing policy of an institution. Individual nurse–patient interactions and nursing policies would then be examined in light of whether they enhanced or negated the principle of respect for both the individual patient and health professional. This principle would apply in all institutions providing services to patients. For example, if a patient told a nurse that she or he did not want a specific treatment, under a principle of respect for the individual, the nurse would not use coercion to force the patient to accept the treatment but would inform the physician of the situation and look at the total pattern of this patient's care and treatment and the meaning of her or his illness and treatment to the patient. Often a patient's refusal of a specific treatment simply gains the individual the label of being a "difficult patient." No health professional currently has an institutionalized responsibility for looking at a given behavior with the patient to determine why the patient is refusing a treatment and what the refusal means to and for the patient's present and future status, for example, increased pain or lack of control over one's own body. The nurse who is the recipient of such information as a request to be allowed to die is in a unique position to assure that this request is not expressed in a void but in an environment of careful listening and following through, as painful as this might be for the nurse. This raises the question as to whose responsibility it is to provide an atmosphere or a "community" where nurses can do this kind of listening and receive support for following through in a difficult and often threatening situation which is a strain for the nurse because of her own vulnerability as a fellow human whose own values might hold that to reject treatment is *ipso facto* wrong. In spite of this, the nurse has an obligation under an ethic of respect for the individual patient to refrain from intruding on the patient's own uniqueness.

Jonsen and Butler point out that one should consider carefully the consequences of accepting this principle as a general guide to decisions and actions. Acceptance of the principle has consequences for the individual patient, for the health professional(s) involved in the patient's care, and for the institution of care, if not the community. To consider further the meaning of the concept:

> Respect denotes an attitude of appreciation and restraint before the uniqueness of individuals. It implies reluctance to intrude into physical integrity, privacy, or the individual purposes constituting that uniqueness. It commands discretion even when interventions are intended to enhance an individual's uniqueness. It requires serious justification when interventions would invade, restrict or diminish uniqueness. It places a high value upon individual freedom, demanding that limitations of freedom be defended by appeal to such reasons as threat to others or provision for common need.[9]

In other words, nursing decisions and actions must be considered in light of whether they enhance or threaten the uniqueness of the individual patient who refuses a specific treatment, another dimension to be articulated in patient care. However, in discussing the refusal of treatment with the patient, the nurse could appeal to a consideration of the impact of the decision on others, for example, family members, if this is in fact the case in a given individual's situation. Nursing action or non-action is thus justified on the moral basis of whether or not it enhances the uniqueness of the individual rather than on a more legalistic basis of "the doctor's orders."

A principle of respect for the individual also seems on the face of it to imply enhancing uniqueness of the involved nurse as an active and thoughtful decision maker. Nurses and patients are both viewed as respected members of the patient-care community. Patients would also be viewed within some recognized limits of safety as active participants in decision making if their physical and psychological status permitted such participation rather than be viewed as the passive object of others' decisions. Instead of asking "why" the patient should be allowed to reject treatment, one could ask "why not?"

If nurses and nursing accept respect for the individual as an underlying ethical principle for decisions and actions, the nurse is placed in a unique position as an advocate for the patient's input in any decisions affecting the patient if these are ignored in the generally paternalistic atmosphere of many hospitals and other health care settings. It also implies the tempering of an extreme position on the traditional medical ethic which says that one should do all one can to preserve an individual's life if the terminally ill patient is receiving treatment in a traditional "cure" setting.

Compassion as a Value

We are *all,* nurses, physicians, patients, judges, and legislators, participating as risk takers in systems and networks where behavior patterns and values are more often ambiguous than sharp and clear. But available technologies need not dictate decision making in any given situation, for example, a particular chemotherapeutic protocol is available so it is automatically used without individual consideration. Can we somehow recognize, articulate, and re-focus on our connectedness and interpersonal responsibilities as members of various communities and on respect for individual freedom and self-determination? Both elements are necessary in making choices around ethical dilemmas in health care. Accepting or rejecting treatment for one's self is only one example. The *process* of compassionate, collaborative decision making in the nurse–physician–patient system and all other system levels involves some conscious, articulate reconciliation of these values. The expression of compassion seems to provide the dynamic link between the values of individual self-determination and interpersonal responsibility as a community member. As Rollo May says, "Compassion is the awareness that we are all in the same boat and that we all shall either sink or swim together."[10] In other words, individuals share each other's joy and pain if they have not become automatons in roles created by and perpetuated in some bureaucracies like the cold, cynical, machine-like nurse.

A compassionate decision making process, with and for suffering individuals, offers all involved the opportunity to articulate and express the value of respect for the individual in a community of caring for both the suffering individual and for those involved and affected by the decision. Nurses, physicians, and family members also suffer in this kind of decision making, which is always tinged with tragedy and a very real sense of our limitations as caring individuals in spite of or perhaps because of our sophisticated technologies. The right to reject treatment *should* take into consideration the consequences of such decisions to the patient's "significant others." One can, at least, argue that these consequences should be considered in the many decisions along the road to the decision about acceptance or rejection of a specific treatment or protocol.

Nurses and nursing are often in a position to influence directly the *process* of decision making and, thus, indirectly the outcomes of the process—a crucial position! Active consideration and thoughtful reflection on respect for both the individual patient and health worker as an underlying ethical principle for nursing could make a difference in how the nursing profession uses this position to make changes in caring for individuals in any setting where nursing is required. Compassionate decision making requires nothing less to enhance the values of respect for the individual and of community.

Endnotes

1. N. K. Brown, J. T. Donovan, R. J. Bulger, and E. H. Laws, "How Do Nurses Feel About Euthanasia and Abortion?" *American Journal of Nursing* 71 (1971), pp. 1415–16.
2. J. Rawls, *A Theory of Justice* (Cambridge, Mass.: Harvard University Press, 1971), pp. 131–135.
3. R. Veatch, "Models for Ethical Medicine in a Revolutionary Age," *Hastings Center Report* 2 (June 1972), p. 5.
4. P. Ramsey, *The Patient as Person* (New Haven: Yale University Press, 1970), p. 133.
5. *Ibid.*, p. 134.
6. Milton Mayeroff, *On Caring* (New York: Harper and Row, 1971), pp. 41–2.
7. Elizabeth Douvan, "The Caring Society," *Educational Horizons* 57 (Fall 1978), pp. 3–9.
8. A. Jonsen and L. Butler, "Public Ethics and Policy Making," *Hastings Center Report* 5 (August 1975), p. 25.
9. *Ibid.*, p. 26.
10. R. May, *Power and Innocence* (New York: Dell, 1972), p. 251.

SECTION

IV

Issues in the Nurse-Patient Relationship

Ours is an age that has been given many names. Prominent among them are references to drugs, to behavior modification, and to manipulation. We have been called, for example, a pill-popping culture—and for good reason. Day and night we are barraged with commercials extolling the miraculous benefits to be gained from a given drug. These drugs range from caffein-laden soft drinks, alcoholic beverages, and patent medicines, to so-called miracle drugs which are understood by doctors alone and which promise cure from a host of serious diseases. We expect to receive drugs to induce sleep or to prevent it, to keep us alert or to ease us into a benign forgetfulness. What is the responsibility of the nurse and the nursing profession in this drug-oriented society?

We live as well in an age of increasing expertise in the matter of modifying the behavior of other persons into patterns we find more congenial and less threatening. Administration of certain types of drugs immeasurably simplifies the often impossibly demanding task of dealing with disoriented or self-threatening individuals. What should the nurse and the nursing profession do when asked or ordered to administer such behavior-modifying agents?

Although ours is an age of the development of technologically sophisticated machinery for the care and treatment of serious and chronic illnesses, it is also an age of scarce resources in these areas. The success of creating such technological advances brings with it the problem of determining to whom such devices will be made available. Is the nurse to remain indifferent to the moral problem presented here or is she obligated by her professional status to develop and to articulate a position consistent with the goals of her profession?

It is not surprising that with a constituency so addicted to the efficiency, presumed or real, of drugs doctors would find the ancient if not honorable practice of prescribing placebos irresistible. Should nurses docilely go along with the practice of giving patients pills which are, in fact, nothing but colored, sugared water? Is there a moral problem here for a professional person? Perhaps there is no problem for someone who does not see herself as a professional, but for a person aspiring to and fulfilling the obligations of a profession, it is clearly a matter of genuine moral and ethical concern when patients are knowingly tricked by their physicians into thinking they are receiving real medicine.

The essays in this section deal with these issues and offer constructive suggestions for the practice of nursing as a humane profession.

Is there a universally accepted principle that applies to all cases in which the nurse is involved in the moral problem of deciding what to do with regard to administering drugs to patients? Elizabeth Maloney offers in this essay an approach to this difficult problem which avoids categorical statements. She insists instead upon a thoughtful consideration of the moral and ethical issues involved in each individual case with which the nurse deals. She argues that very basic issues of conscience are found in the context of determining the nurse's proper approach to drug administration. Sensitivity to these moral concerns is central to the appropriate response of the nursing professional as Maloney presents it.

II

Doctors, Nurses, and Drugs: Notes on the Meaning and Ethics of Administration

Elizabeth M. Maloney

Once, those of us who elected careers in the health field also elected a calling. The heart of that "calling" was a loose consensus on what constituted professional ethics. In the education of health workers, sometimes it was as concrete as a course in a program of study; always at the end it was an oath or a pledge to summarize and seal the promise for the future. The word dedication has fallen into disrepute to be replaced by chi squared and contingency—as technology, zero-based budgeting, and union contracts replace "calling." In part rightly so, for there is little question but that the very dedication was frequently exploited. The demand for around-the-clock service to humanity was an unreal and dehumanizing expectation in some institutions. It has been replaced by a more professionalized stance, which has as one of its implicit tenets that loyalty to an institution is, more often than not, loyalty misplaced. It is to the clients of the institution or practice—*raison d'etre* of each—that allegiance is owed. Advocacy movements which have gained so much ground in the past decade are, in part, recognition of how far we have drifted away from the calling and, second, they are rational attempts not to replace technology but to surround it with operational humanistic encounters.

Gaylin has noted that in the last twenty years swift developments in science have "precipitated a whole new dialogue on ethical and value issues."[1] There is no doubt that this is so. Centers have been established to conduct these dialogs. A thematic analysis of the literature leads quite simply to the observation that this whole "humanistic" movement in medicine, medical schools, nursing, and nursing education is, in part, an attempt to replace what was once called the "art" of medical healing or nursing care. It is also an attempt to strike a new balance between technology and the people who must use it, both staff and patients. For the two revolutions, therapeutic and technological, are artifacts of our own century. Lenihan points out that:

> It is not always appreciated that the first man-made drug (if we exclude anaesthetics) was aspirin, which did not leave the factory till 1899. Since then we have seen the successive triumphs of chemotherapy in sulpho-namides, antibiotics and tranquilizers.[2]

The two revolutions, or their aftermath, have often blended to make one stream. It is uncommon to have an ethical question emerge in the care of the terminally ill where both drugs and life-supporting technology are not simultaneously at issue.

It is against this backdrop that drugs and medications will be discussed. The health professional-institutional culture and the larger culture merge to consti-tute attitudes, beliefs, and actions that motivate drug giving and drug consump-tion in the interests of the relief of human suffering.

There are, perhaps, an even dozen activities performed by health professionals that act as symbols in the public mind. These symbolic acts are the stuff of real life, but become symbolic as they are played out over and over again on tele-vision screens, motion pictures, and in novels. Just to name a few in passing, they are: resuscitation of the suddenly stricken, administration of life saving substances either by oral medication or injection . . . and the figures in white constantly referring to electronic monitoring devices. Less dramatic are the everyday occasions when we first turn to our own private network of self-help, and only when that fails do we turn to professional help. For as one physician has noted about health in the United States, "No one takes public note of the truth of the matter, which is that most people in this country have a clear, unimpeded run at a longer life-time than could be foreseen by any earlier genera-tion."[3] Parenthetically, then, it can be said that one almost always tries other routes before approaching the professional whether the problem is legal, med-ical, or other.[4] In reference to the consumption of non-prescription drugs, most of us "dose" for various things, as well as consult the stars, the neighbors, and the newspaper health columns for insight into our malaise.

Self-Dosage and Prescribed Drugs

The populace in every country has firm conceptions about drugs. There are those used for occasions when people have discomfort, formulate their view of the cause, and take some non-prescription drug for an expected effect. These clearly codified perceptions apparently emerge gradually in the culture from a variety of sources and are modified through observation and experience in families, peer groups, and through instruments of the larger culture, such as television and other advertisements.

One study found that while most first graders do not have too clear an idea of what drugs are, most third graders involved had "a good idea" of what drugs are.[5] Certainly non-prescription drugs are often identified for rather specific symptoms such as stomach upsets and headaches (frequently accompanied by graphics purporting to indicate speed of pain relief for trapped gas or tension headaches). Since there is a definite cluster of these advertised symptoms, complete with stated limits and warnings, certainly those symptoms *not* described constitute, by their absence, another group for which a more formalized relief is sought through physicians and prescriptive drugs. For example, double vision and fainting episodes are not symptoms that are discussed in the media. Therefore, there would appear to be some rough rule of thumb related to self-diagnosis and self-prescription of drugs in the culture. Apparently self-diagnosis and self-prescription partially serve the purpose of avoiding the formal health care system as long as it is feasible or possible.

Probably a distinction now needs to be made (or a line drawn) between those agents which belong in the permissible self-dosage area and those clearly in the prescribed arena. A third large category of drugs is addictive substances and for purposes of limiting the scope of this discussion, only the self-dosage and the legally prescribed drugs will be dealt with here. These drugs encompass any substance that can be ingested, either liquid or solid, injectables, vapors, unguents, and various embrocations. The foregoing constitute a wide array of avenues for introducing substances into the human body for relief of real or perceived maladies.

Paradoxically there are some substances that are so much a part of the household that they are not viewed as drugs; yet these same substances may be prescribed as part of a treatment regimen in a hospital setting. The most common illustration is aspirin. Prescribed in five or more grains on a hospital order sheet, it is also self-administered for self-defined ailments. Clearly a great deal depends on the definition of the setting and situation by a particular agent. Vitamins of all kinds can be included in this general group as well. Gebhardt, Governali, and Hart found about 77 percent of a sample of senior citizens "believed that all older people should take vitamins."[6] In one recent year, more than four hundred million dollars were spent for vitamins.

It is always instructive and necessary to examine the semantics of any profession. The language we learn and use in many ways limits our perception and control of the world. Our ability to engage in abstract thought, to name, define, and limit a situation is also closely connected with the number of options we have available to deal with a given problem. It is probably no accident that military language or the language of warfare appears in reference to the control of some illnesses—bodies are invaded by disease; we fight off illnesses; and, as has been pointed out recently, treatment of cancer has associated with it

terminology straight from the language of war. Patients are "bombarded" with
targeted rays, we make "war" on cancer,[7] and comment is made about Erlich's
"magic bullet" as early as the year 1910. In one of a series of three articles
recently published Sontag considers the words *shoot* and *shot,* respectively
verb and noun, to describe the injectable administration of a drug.[8] This is now
so commonplace a description for hypodermic medication, in the vernacular at
least, that no one ever thinks about it any more. So much is it used that it has
leaked over into the professional lexicon, at least when communicating to
selected patients. Carrying it one step forward, in the argot of the streets,
addicts shoot up; a collection of drug users in their place of activity is often
characterized (in part) by the segment of professional workers engaged in
relieving drug addiciton, for example, as busy in a "shooting gallery." This is
the military language of the street. Thus, it can be said that part of the old
professional calling, now the new humanism, is to make war on disease. One
of the powerful weapons that humanistic physicians and nurses have in their
arsenals is drugs. Without forcing the campaign analogy further, we can speculate
that many persons who enlist in the war against disease hate to lose. As in any
conflict, ethical and moral questions about procedure are frequently met, since
the outcome of any war has grave consequences for all of the participants. It
is interesting, whether or not it is significant, that some of the activities undertaken in the name of care and cure are couched in the language of the cam-
paigner. Whether or not this occurs with more frequency than in the general
speech of every day or of specific enclaves in any culture is open for discussion. The next step will be to examine the role drugs and medications play
in relieving pain and in bolstering the professional self-image—for as surely as
one is possible, so is the other.

Relief of Pain and the Promise of Cure: Professional Power and Drugs

It has been noted frequently that pain is part of the human condition. The
world's literature is full of eloquently expressed examples of humanity's physical
and psychological pain—and the efforts to relieve it. Science and technology
have offered answers in recent years[9] and among the most frequently used
methods for the relief of pain are drugs. In the realm of cure or respite from
disease, spectacular relief from a large number of formerly lethal and crippling
diseases has been made. So much so that the expectations of the American
people have risen to an unprecedented level.[10] An example illustrates this
point. Once every county and city, as well as many states, had a specialized system of institutions for the care of those persons with tuberculosis. Whole towns
grew up as partial support systems for these institutions (Saranac comes to mind,
for one). The discovery of an effective and specific drug for this disease has
largely shut these hospital systems down. It has also eliminated a once rich

source for novelistic interpretation of tragedy for individuals. Mann's *Magic Mountain* is an example. As one of the illnesses with particular impact on the public mind as a destroyer of persons, it has largely been displaced by cancer.[11] (The latter is simply viewed as a destroyer. There is none of the romantic wasting away of tuberculosis with this disease.) Nonetheless, having found what appear to be specifics for polio prevention, control of diabetes, and other human ailments, the class of professional who is privy to these and other magic-like drugs is very powerful indeed.

Primum Non Nocere—*First, Do No Harm*

It might be instructive to look briefly at the way the neophyte in one of the health professions learns to handle drugs, not from the viewpoint of didactic learning but from the vantage point of custom, "atrocity or horror" story, the impact of exhortation and ritual upon how drugs are handled and by whom— in short, a brief reference to the hospital drug culture.

First, it should be noted that safety, exactness, and addiction are the triple themes generated in the clinical culture. To provide safety and exactness of administration, there is ritual and rule—check three times or the rule of three; the atrocity story has to do with the perpetration of error and the graphic, word of mouth description of the mistake and its subsequent punishment in the hospital world. All of this exerts a powerful pull on the behavior of those administering drugs, since the possibility of error and ethical dilemma are built into the situation.

The placing of blame in any organization is an interesting phenomenon. Sometimes it is directly related to failure to perform a function or set of functions; for example, a drug is not given. According to one recent source "omitted dosage accounts for about a third of all the mistakes in giving drugs," approximately 37 percent of all errors.[12] Since the general run of omission and comission errors is made without initial awareness of the mistake, the ethical questions arise first in the area of reporting—self-reporting or reporting others when error is identified. The latter is a particularly loaded area. As difficult as it might be to acknowledge one's own error, the situation intensifies when others are involved, particularly if the context includes a probable degree of harm to the patient. There are so many factors, degrees of possible culpability, and at least three major perspectives from which such ethical considerations may be examined. Carlton examines the "primacy of clinical judgment over moral choice."[13]

There are two potential lines of error in the administration of drugs. These lines are related directly to role. Physicians prescribe and, not surprisingly, if errors are made, they tend to be in either the area of unsafe dosages or some modification in the orthodox administration of the substance. Nurses administer drugs and in that act provide the structure for infinite possibilities of error— and the accompanying blame. It is necessary to note that nurses are not the only ones giving drugs; however, they still administer the vast majority of drugs given. Physicians are the sole group legally authorized to write prescriptions for drugs. No one else except dentists can do this, and their repertoire is characteristically circumscribed by comparison. (There is also a small group of physician's assistants who are beginning to write specific types of orders, but there are many nurses reluctant or refusing altogether to honor such efforts.)

The very human temptation to avoid blame and the ensuing discomfort and the typical hospital structure militate in an hierarchical fashion against at least one class of mistakes being freely exposed. It has been amply documented that physicians exert the primary power in situations where drugs are administered. Physicians have been known to argue for the administration of a dose twice a drug's safe amount and some institutions have developed policies for nursing staff to enable them to refuse participation. Much more difficult to detect are the nursing errors which, while they remain unreported, lead physicians to make false assumptions about progress or lack of progress with a given patient. This whole, complex situation has changed and will change further as an increasing number of institutions employ the unit-dose system of drug distribution. Since under this system the pharmacist packages the drug and the nurse administers it, at very least they will be jointly held liable for error, for whatever comfort that brings either group.

The knottiest problems of all remain matters of individual conscience or ethical responsibility in juxtaposition to the urgencies and pressures of daily life in the hospital and clinical situation. Carlton argues that academic efforts to provide ethical training for physicians in medical schools must somehow surmount the gap between the classroom and the clinical arena.[14] Closely allied to this is a situation in the education of nursing students described by Newton and Newton.[15] Briefly, when asked to respond to an hypothetical problem where a doctor telephoned orders for twice the usual dosage of an unfamiliar drug, nearly all students were able to provide justification for not carrying out the order. Twenty-one out of twenty-two nurses in active practice, however, were ready to accept the order over the telephone. In this one cited instance, it would seem that some sort of on-the-spot clinical judgment had been made. The basis of this judgment was probably somehow detached from academic, ethical factors. The authors describing the example felt that "nurses must be living within a professional double standard."[16] In theory, there is one answer; in practice another style prevails. This gap deserves further study.

Placebo—*I Shall Please*

Most of the practitioners in the health field are introduced to the administration of the placebo through the informal clinical practice system and very rarely indeed through formal classes related to pharmacology. In fact, it is an area almost never developed in textbooks, except in invective against it as a dubious procedure.

A placebo is basically a false medication—an imposter drug masquerading, for the patient at least, as the genuine article. There are two situations in which the placebo may emerge as a solution to a clinical problem. The patient usually complains persistently of pain or inability to sleep (frequently in tandem) to nursing and medical staff. At first, all effort is extended to locate the difficulty. In time, the conclusion that there is no organic reason for the "complaint" is reached. Is there, then, a clear recognition that a psychological difficulty is at the base of the difficulty? Psychological problems may be assumed as manifest or implicit, and administration of tranquilizers is not uncommon. In fact, it can be postulated that the use of placebo has diminished in direct proportion to the proliferation of these drugs. One is much less likely to complain when viewing the hospital world through a pink haze of chemical. The tranquilizer can be a placebo when it is offered to the patient under the guise of a solution to an irrational, unfounded complaint; a serendipitous payload all to the good. The second quality or characteristic related to administration of the placebo is the persistence or sheer nuisance value of the patient's behavior. If the volume and mode of complaint stretches the level of tolerance of a given group of health workers, the likelihood of placebo administration increases in proportion to the perceived powerlessness of the staff to deal directly and effectively with the problem.

If the injection of sterile water, or whatever, "works" there is usually at least a modicum of levity among the staff. For the time being, the problem is settled. Perhaps it is even settled for good, particularly since hospital stays tend to be short in these days. Psychologically engendered problems have a way of returning, however, either in the same or other forms. This tends to render the placebo a palliative, particularly in long-term care situations.

Assuming there are times when the advantages of the placebo outweigh the disadvantages, there are ethics involved for those who care to consider them. Essentially, proffering an ersatz medication to a patient is cashing in on the trust that individual has invested in the situation. Bok has described the practice of giving placebos as illustrating: ". . . two miscalculations so common to minor forms of deceit, ignoring possible harm and failing to see how gestures assumed to be trivial build up into collectively undesirable practice."[17]

Since nurses are almost always the agents of administration, their willingness to participate in the administration of placebos probably has to be considered on a case-by-case basis. All the more so because it is the complaints of nursing personnel, anchored in the patient's environment twenty-four hours a day, that frequently influence physicians to prescribe for the nurses' rather than the patient's relief. That is not to say that some situations do not reach impasses where placebos are relatively benevolent solutions, for, regrettable as it may seem, that is the case. As Bok says, "this is not to say that all placebos must be ruled out; merely that they cannot be excused as innocuous."[18]

It is instructive to look at advertisements for drugs as they are presented to physicians. Since mood altering drugs are among those whose success gains the most gratitude for the helping professional, it is likely that the search for more refined, useful, misery-relieving drugs will go on. One way to keep abreast is to read the professional journals and their proposals—with the caveat that these messages are directed to experienced readers.

A few of the more picturesque are:

A middle aged woman is present full face; she is clearly weeping, distressed, and depressed. In bold type, this message: "you can promise her that she'll improve tonight."

A man, head bowed, standing waist high in a wheat field; he is alone and it is sunset. Caption: "Hopelessness and isolation are cutting him off from life." Below, the product and its full description, complete with side effects.

"Put depression safely behind them." In this one, a man and woman, hand in hand, stride briskly toward the reader, full face.

Since it is highly unlikely that a prescription will be written on the basis of the foregoing, what purpose does advertising serve? Particularly since many of the accompanying drug descriptions are straightforward, is it possible to elicit at least a promise implicit in some of these captions? For depressions are widespread and they are sometimes difficult to deal with, as are many other psychiatric conditions. A thematic analysis of this type of advertising might turn up a statement such as "power for the powerless healer."

Patients who do not take their medication are subjects of exasperation and concern to physicians and nurses alike.[19] Although both nurses and physicians agree with Cousins that "one of the main functions of the doctor is to engage to the fullest the patient's own ability to mobilize the forces of mind and body in turning back disease,"[20] taking prescribed drugs is part of the mobilization.

One of the patient's prime responsibilities is to cooperate in every way, and that includes taking ordered medications. There are occasions where failure to do so is to court self-destruction—a time worn example is the diabetic and insulin. There are less dramatic instances where the consequences are not as lethal and where failure to take medications sometimes is reduced to a power-powerless situation between professional and patient. Part of the professional's exasperation is then at bottom powerlessness to control the situation or to exert leverage on the illness.

Nurses have their own problems with this situation. In addition to all of the loss of control or omnipotence, they also loose face as a persuader. For it is still a given in the hospital setting that orders are made to be carried out. At best, the nurse is held to lack the ability to persuade if a patient refuses medication. This is not unique to nursing practice in institutions; it is similar to public school teachers and refusal of a given child to maintain decorum in a classroom. (In hierarchical situations in the United States, leadership is in part the ability to persuade.) Once the misbehavior is recognized outside the individual nurse-patient situation or the child–teacher pairing, an unofficial, group label is affixed (uncooperative) and the practitioner's ability is no longer in question. The onus rests on the client—"they do not want to get well."[21] Applebaum adds that reasons given for refusing one's medication can be thought of as resistance or as a defense against anxiety,[22] but not taking your medication is a cardinal sin in the hospital world.

Administration of Drugs as Coercion

In the usual sense of the word, coercion implies threat or fear and Gaylin notes that humans are uniquely able to anticipate and imagine and to respond to very subtle degrees of coercion.[23] To be more specific, because of "the finiteness of life and the fragility of existence, man is uniquely equipped to be coerced."[24]

In a broad sense, children are civilized into a culture by the process of praise and blame, blame being viewed as psychologically coercive in this context.[25] The field of medicine ranks next to parents in "enjoying wide institutional privileges of coercion."[26] It is only necessary to recall quarantine of ships, families, and individuals, or the legal commitment of persons to mental hospitals, to come to the conclusion that certain forms of illness are threat enough to the whole to legalize incarceration of the part or the individual. The use of restraints and physical force in hospitals and prisons has historically been thought of as for the good of the whole. Force, then, can bind or constrict an individual physically, but it can also be applied psychologically to influence motivation and behavior, particularly by health professionals who have the weight of expertise on their side in life-threatening situations.

If a patient with advanced cancer decides to discontinue chemotherapy, for example, because the side effects are destroying the quality of the life she or he has left to live, it takes conviction on the patient's part to withstand professional sanctions and pressures to continue medications.

The prescription of a drug by a physician can be a statement of medical knowledge and subsequent treatment of an identified condition. Halleck identifies the prescription of drugs as a significant social statement.[27] The individual's problem is identified as being within her- or himself as opposed to outside; the individual is now sick and the sick in particular take pills. In the years since their discovery in the early 1950s the widespread use and abuse of tranquilizers, sedatives, and, in due course, anti-depressants, has had considerable impact on the way people view difficulties in life. In 1969, approximately 700,000 pounds of barbiturates were marketed, that is thirty doses a year for each of us.[28] There were fifty types of sedatives and barbiturates then and the number has multiplied since. Some or all of these drugs have been given to psychiatric patients, frequently without their willing cooperation and often over a considerable span of time. Since no one yet knows what effect the long-term administration of massive doses of thorazine, for example, on an individual will be, what are the ethics of administration? Complaints from patients about fuzziness, about all degrees of discomfort in living are frequently heard. Yet would these people be able to function at all in some areas without the drug? The morality of chemical control over one set of individuals (patients) by another (health professionals) is at this time a razor sharp balancing act of one set of arguments and data against another. It is the unthinking conviction that one has the truth about the matter because one is a professional that may be the ethical lapse and the point at issue. At any rate the law, which has long recognized that coercion need not involve physical force,[29] is being invoked with growing skill by organizations of former mental patients. In an area such as health coercion has been built in, particularly in regard to many of the treatments for the mentally ill. By placing the disturbed behavior of a large number of people within a medical frame, we have legitimized the coercive administration of mood-changing drugs.

In terms of nursing administration, particularly of prescribed drugs for the relief of pain, there are two areas which deserve examination. One is the relatively unexplored area of just how and what kind of nursing care would reduce the continued administration of narcotics and other drugs. In some general hospitals, almost everyone on a given unit gets a sleeping pill every night until and including the night prior to discharge. The second question is the belief of the professional in the efficacy of the drug being administered. Certainly if a staff is dealing with a new drug that they view as particularly specific and powerful this aura of belief communicates to the recipient in some undefinable fashion. Minimally at least, it contributes to well-being in the maximization of hope in the patient— in and of itself a potent healing force. Related to the foregoing is the placebo and the placebo effect. As a recent source has indicated, giving placeboes, however benevolent the intent, is a form of lying.[30]

A survey of nursing efforts to relieve pain by means other than drugs indicates activities which include a range of the following, dependent on the condition involved in each case: repositioning following surgery, pre- and post-operative support including visits from personnel, communication, giving the patient a sense of control, and the like.[31]

There has always appeared to be a shadow of irrationality in the way drugs are administered to the dying. Now and again an instance is located where there seems to be an underlying concern about addicting people who are dying and who, furthermore, are dying in severe pain. It would seem irrational here to automatically administer drugs according to the clock.

There is an excellent model which has developed for the control of pain in the hospices, many of whose elements can be adapted for other usage. Many, *not* all, since the oral medication, for example, known as Brompton's Mixture (used in St. Christopher's in London) contained cocaine. It has been modified for use in this country and, in two instances, legal dispensation for the use of heroin have been sanctioned.

However, the aim of controlling pain while maintaining alertness means development of an effective system of pain control[32] and that turns out to be not as much what is in the medication as how and when it is given. The fear of pain increases the pain and one of the hospices initiated a comfort chart kept by the patients—who also dispense and administer their own medication.[33]

Summary

Reliance on drugs to take the edge from problems has become a commonplace of existence, at least among certain groups of people. Necessary to the hospital-illness culture, a set of attitudes which largely falls in the realm of the slightly out-of-awareness pervades the giver of medication and the taker. All of us have developed an inordinate faith that if the machine breaks down, we can swallow the remedy. Or if there isn't one, we loose confidence in the huge health system and those who are associated with it. It is, after all "a system that bestows enormous power on those who control it."[34]

Individuals seem to have less and less assurance that they can control their environment and have turned over some of the aspects of health to others. There are heartening signs that people are interested in prevention, but there are still too many who continue to feel that, if you live dangerously, an all-powerful health system is standing by to administer the relieving drug and apply the technology to replace the organ.

Too often in medicine and in other areas, both dollars and priorities have been directed toward picking up the pieces, instead of preventing the fall.[35]

Endnotes

1. Willard Gaylin, "On the Borders of Persuasion: A Psychoanalytic Look at Coercion," *Psychiatry* 37, no. 1 (February 1974), pp. 1-9.
2. John Lenihan, "Technology or TLC: The Nurse's Dilemma," *Nursing Times* (August 1977), p. 1266.
3. Lewis Thomas, "On the Science and Technology of Medicine," *Daedalus* 106, no. 9 (Winter 1977), p. 43.
4. Martin Bloom, *The Paradox of Helping* (New York: Wiley, 1975).
5. James Korn, "The Concept of a Drug in First and Third Grade Children," *Journal of Drug Education* 8, no. 1 (1978), pp. 59-67.
6. Mary Gebhardt, Joseph Governali, and Edward Hart, "Drug-Related Behavior, Knowledge and Misconceptions Among a Selected Group of Senior Citizens," *Journal of Drug Education* 8, no. 2 (1978), pp. 85-92.

7. Daniel Greenberg, "The War on Cancer: Official Fiction and Harsh Fact," *Science and Governmental Report* 4 (December 1974).
8. Susan Sontag, "The Political Language of Disease," *The New York Review* 25, no. 2 (February 1978), p. 30.
9. Jeanne Benoliel, "Foreword," in *Pain: A Source Book for Nurses and Other Health Professionals,* ed. Ada Jacoz (Boston: Little, Brown, 1977).
10. John Knowles, "Doing Better and Feeling Worse: Health in the United States," *Daedalus* 106, no. 9 (Winter 1977), p. 4.
11. Susan Sontag, "Images of Illness," *The New York Review* 25, no. 1 (February 1978), p. 27.
12. Marion Newton and David Newton, "Guidelines for Handling Drug Errors," *Nursing 77* (September), p. 64.
13. Wendy Carlton, *In Our Professional Opinion . . .* (Notre Dame, Ind.: University of Notre Dame Press, 1979).
14. *Ibid.*
15. Newton and Newton, "Guidelines for Handling Drug Errors."
16. *Ibid.,* p. 64.
17. Sissela Bok, *Lying: Moral Choice and Private Life* (New York: Pantheon, 1978), p. 61.
18. *Ibid.,* p. 68.
19. Greenberg, "The War on Cancer."
20. Norman Cousins, "What I Learned from 3,000 Doctors," *Saturday Review of Literature* 5, no. 10 (February 1978), p. 12.
21. Stephen A. Applebaum, "The Refusal to Take One's Medicine," *Bulletin of the Menninger Clinic* 41, no. 6 (November 1977), p. 511.
22. *Ibid.*
23. W. Gaylin, "On the Boundaries of Persuasion," p. 1.
24. *Ibid.,* p. 5.
25. Harry Stack Sullivan, *The Interpersonal Theory of Psychiatry* (New York: W. W. Norton, 1953).
26. Gaylin, "On the Boundaries of Persuasion," p. 5.
27. Seymour Halleck, *The Politics of Therapy* (New York: Harper and Row, 1971).
28. Elton B. McNeil, *Human Socialization* (Belmont, Cal.: Brooks/Cole Publishing, 1969).
29. Gaylin, "On the Boundaries of Persuasion," p. 3.
30. Bok, *Lying.*
31. Ada Jacox, ed., *Pain: A Source Book for Nurses and Other Health Professionals* (Boston: Little, Brown, 1977).
32. Sandol Stoddard, *The Hospice Movement* (New York: Briarcliff Manor, Stein and Day, 1978), pp. 48–49.
33. *Ibid.*
34. Marc La Londe, "The Canadian Health Care System: Its Impact on the Health of the Society," in *Medicine in a Changing Society* (St. Louis: C. V. Mosby, 1977).
35. Edward Kennedy, "Legislative Realities in National Health Insurance," in *Medicine in a Changing Society* (St. Louis: C. V. Mosby, 1977).

In this essay Jay Schulkin and Robert Neville further develop the moral and ethical issues of drug administration by focusing on the particularly problematic matter of the treatment of mental patients with behavior-changing drugs. Theirs is a carefully reasoned essay built upon moral principles which we see as basic to the nursing profession throughout this book. These principles are that persons ought to be free and responsible—patients and nurses alike—and that society and its institutions should do everything within their power to safeguard the first principle of individual freedom and individual responsibility. While few would be disposed to argue against such moral principles, the problems arise as soon as one leaves the area of philosophical abstraction and enters the real world, so to speak, of the hospital and, more particularly, the wards that house patients too ill to exercise their moral right of freedom and responsibility. This essay makes clear that nurses do not operate alone, but in a complex setting in which decisions are made which involve not only nurses but also doctors and, in one way or another, the social order itself through its appointed representatives in governmental agencies and institutional policy-makers.

12

Responsibility, Rehabilitation, and Drugs: Health Care Dilemmas

Jay Schulkin and Robert Neville

Psychotropic drugs uniquely alter a person's relation to the world. Whatever their pleasures or benefits, they reinforce dependence, either in the ways they operate or in the social relations involved in their use. Psychotropic drugs, therefore, pose striking dilemmas of responsibility and authority and of individual *versus* social goods.

Some of these dilemmas can be sorted out by examining psychotropic drugs in two contexts. The first is the treatment of psychotropic (more precisely, opiate) drug abusers. The second is the treatment of mental patients with psychotropic drugs.

Teasing out certain crucial moral elements in each of these contexts, specific policy recommendations will be made. The recommendations themselves, however, rest in part on two general moral principles that may be mentioned here and illustrated in what follows. Although both deserve a more complete articulation and defense than is possible here, they shall be stated here as if they present values generally agreed upon by those who reflect.

The first principle is that persons ought to be free and responsible. Three conditions obtain if a person is responsible.

First, the person is in a position to make a difference to situations for better or worse. The scope of the person's responsibilities is the range of situations in which it is casually possible for that person to affect things for the better or worse.

Second, the person must be able to adopt the better course for reasons of its perceived value; this refers to potentialities in the person's character. The person must be able to be aware of the value of the better course, for instance, in order to be able to adopt it *for its worth*. For drug addicts and mental patients, the relevant impediment to responsibility is that their mental disorder might make it impossible for them to be able to adopt the better course, especially where better course means the "right decision" regarding medication.

A person *has* responsibilities regarding those situations that he or she can influence for better or worse and where the person *can* make the choice with reference to the distinction between better and worse. This is to have responsibilities and be responsible. But to *fulfill* responsibilities, to take responsibility, to behave responsibly is a different matter. That a person *can* choose the better does not entail that he or she *will* choose the better. A person should not only have responsibilities but also fulfill them as an autonomous agent. Hence, the third condition of responsibility is that a person should have the character, skills, and habits of generally fulfilling responsibility.

The distinction between having responsibilities, defined by the first two conditions, and fulfilling them generally, defined by the third, is crucial. Whether or not a person fulfills responsibilities is a moral matter, not one of scientific feasibility. A person who is capable of exercising responsibility and fails is immoral, irresponsible, or simply mistaken, not incapable of responsibility or in need of someone else to make the decision. The major question about mental patients and addicts, however, sometimes seems to be whether they are in fact capable of making responsible decisions, not whether they make the right decisions.

There is a special complication here. The capacity to behave responsibly is developed in small increments, and it is learned through the very exercise of making choices and being held responsible for them. This is obviously true of children who become responsible through being given responsibilities in ever-widening areas, while not being held responsible in areas outside their capacities. It is also true, most likely, with adult mental patients. While incapable of the full range of adult responsibilities, they may be capable of small areas of responsibility, and restoration of the full range requires the exercise of increasing responsibility in small increments.

This leads to the second principle. Society and its institutions should foster personal freedom and responsibility by demanding it of everyone, teaching it where possible, and rewarding it, all at the various appropriate levels. Children should be taught responsibilities in increments appropriate to their age and learning capacities. This is the justifiable rationale behind compulsory schooling. Adults too should be aided and reinforced in and held accountable for taking responsibility.

We usually make an important distinction between children and adults, however. With regard to children the obligation of society is to foster not only the capacity to have responsibilities but also the habits and character of fulfilling them, on the grounds that the practice of fulfilling a restricted range of responsibilities is necessary for developing the potential to have responsibilities of an adult range. For instance, society has an obligation to insist not only that children be able to learn but that they in fact learn, because if they remain ignorant or unskilled in certain crucial areas they will not be capable of having certain adult responsibilities. With regard to adults, however, society has the obligation to insist with pressure only that they be capable of acting responsibly, not that they in fact fulfill their responsibilities. If they do not fulfill their responsibilities we hold them morally or criminally liable. Being held morally accountable is a central element of human dignity. Even children should be held accountable in areas where they have developed the capacity for responsibility.

With these two principles in mind, consider the following problems of responsibility and treatment in the case of abusers of illegal drugs.

II

Ten years after their influential article reporting on the successful use of methadone in the treatment of a small group of intractable heroin addicts, Vincent P. Dole and Marie E. Nyswander stated:

> No medicine can rehabilitate persons. Methadone maintenance makes possible a first step toward social rehabilitation by stabilizing the pharmacological condition of addicts who have been living as criminals on the fringe of society.[1]

The methadone programs developed over the ten years prior to this statement, however, have not provided that first step. Dole and Nyswander went on to say,

> To succeed in bringing disadvantaged addicts to a productive way of life, a treatment must enable its patients to feel pride and hope and to accept responsibility. This is often not achieved in present-day treatment programs. Without mutual respect, an adversary relationship develops between patients and staff, reinforced by arbitrary rules and the indifference of persons in authority. Patients held in contempt by the staff continue to act like addicts, and the overcrowded facility becomes a public nuisance. Understandably, methadone maintenance programs today have little appeal to the communities or to the majority of heroin addicts on the streets.[2]

The criticism of methadone programs calls for basic rethinking of the concept of rehabilitation. For, as they pointed out, "no medicine can rehabilitate persons."

Drug addiction must first of all be seen as dependence on chemicals. The same psychological factors that lead some people to drugs might lead others to different dependencies, for instance religion, work, or sex; but those other dependencies are different from drug addiction and should not be confused with it. The social and economic factors that lead some people to drugs stimulate others to aggressive striving. Rather than obscuring the drug problem by association with all forms of addictive dependency or social alienation, it should be understood initially as a health problem of coping with the addictive chemicals and then as a set of personal and social problems resulting from the use of drugs.

The basic distinguishing marks of opiate addiction in contrast to other, perhaps equally harmful, dependencies are the use and effects of the chemicals. It would be naive to say that the psychological effects of opiate drugs are purely physical functions; the placebo effects, for instance, are too well known. Furthermore, the meanings of the drug and of the feelings for a person's life depend on a great many factors of prior experience and expectations. But there are two kinds of effects that relate very closely to the physical action of the drugs and are best handled as problems of health care: (1) the physical withdrawal symptoms and (2) the positive learned responses to euphoric feelings that reinforce many aspects of the drug life. Persons can stop taking drugs completely and suddenly, or by slowly decreasing doses over a period of time; either way involves some possible physical danger and can be made easier with supervision by medical health care professionals. Regarding the euphoric feelings, medications such as methadone and narcotic antagonists can be given to prevent their occurring, thereby helping to decondition addicts to the pursuit of more drugs at higher dosages. In general, treatments by health care professionals can help stabilize addicts with respect to drugs, either by withdrawing them or by finding a level of maintenance that allows them to face the other problems of the world, including further therapy.

Drug stabilization is usually a condition for further therapy even though it does not go very far toward rehabilitation itself if there are serious reasons, beyond the mere feel of them, addicts take drugs. Although it is difficult to find a model of "disease" in which drug addiction can legitimately be called a disease, at its heart it involves a health care problem.

Therefore, the best way to handle the *health care* aspects of drug addiction is to consider them as health problems to be dealt with by physicians and nurses with the addicts acting in the role of patients. Health care professionals should be allowed to supervise detoxification and physicians should be allowed to prescribe opiates at a maintenance level or at slowly detoxifying levels as seems best for the health of the patient. Furthermore, what course *should* be taken, for instance, withdrawal or maintenance at this level or that, is a matter to be worked out between the health care supervisor and patient, with informed consent observed. The supervisor would indicate the effects of various alternatives, and would operate within limits set by good medical practice (for instance, no methadone maintenance at levels higher than 120 mgs. per day). The heart of this health care model is that the therapeutic goals are the responsibility of the patient.

Some people might respond negatively to the suggestion that addicts in conjunction with the medical professionals be allowed to determine the goals of their treatment. Common sense might suggest that if addicts had taken drugs to secure extreme euphoria or the narcosis of "nodding out," they would continue to choose to do so under medical support.

But they should be allowed to do so, if this case should occur, because not to allow it would be to reinforce their passivity. It is a mistake to act as if the society or professional world knows best how the addict should live, not because the experts may not have more wisdom, but because imposing that wisdom on the addict reinforces the basic dependency. Furthermore, empirical evidence suggests that addicts are responsive themselves to the freedom to engage life without drugs or with moderate levels of drug use. A study by Goldstein, Hansteen, and Horns indicates that when a group of methadone patients were allowed to regulate their dosage (up to a maximum of 120 mg. per day) they did not gravitate to the maximum. Only two out of ninety-nine chose the maximum, and at the end of the experiment three quarters of the population had dosages of 70 mg. or less.[3]

This proposal for medicalizing treatment, which conforms somewhat to the practice in Great Britain and most European countries, would require several changes in the law as it stands in the United States. Most obviously it would require legislation allowing physicians to distribute heroin and other opiates as they do any prescription drugs. For patients who choose it, understanding the health care advantages and disadvantages, opiate maintenance should be considered a way of handling their medical problem.

The social context for the medical stabilization of drug addicts should be the same as for the treatment of any health problems. In middle and upper income social groups this usually means family physicians, perhaps the ideal situation. Family physicians and their staffs are best able to encourage patients to take responsible roles in care of their own health, and can establish personal relationships with patients over time. Lower income groups in the present situation make greater use of clinics and other medical facilities. While these are not optimum for health care in many instances, it is important that the medical aspects of drug addiction be taken care of as one kind of health problem among others. There are several positive reasons for this.

The chief reason for insisting on the medicalization of this aspect of therapy for addicts is *not* to cope with medical dangers or to keep medicines in the hands of physicians; indeed, there are many arguments in other spheres for allowing nurses and paraprofessionals to oversee medical problems and even to dispense opiates as therapeutics. But physicians and their staffs are important here because they can call upon addicts to take responsible roles in the care of their own health.

Of course the paternalism of the medical profession is a general problem in this regard; but there is more dignity in being treated by a doctor, who also treats other aspects of your health and has responsibility for prescription, than in only meeting a nurse whose main job is to dispense opiates. Of course as new roles for nurses give them more responsibility, they take on proportionately greater importance in fostering responsibility in addicts.

Another aspect of responsibility in connection with drug stabilization is that connection with physicians and nurses in a health context greatly lessens the punitive sense of treatment so characteristic of health care in treatment programs aimed at drug addicts. Whatever psychological or moral faults the addicts may have that led them into drugs, and whatever immoral or criminal activity they might engage in as part of the drug life, those are *not* concerns of the health care professionals. Rather their concern is for providing help in stabilizing the addicts' physical use of drugs. This factor has the advantage of incorporating the addicts more willingly in the beginning stages of taking care of themselves.

One of the chief drawbacks to drug clinics *per se,* whatever their therapeutic modality, is that they collect people interested in drugs; many clinics have become prime "connection" points. In contrast, the clientel of a family physician or health clinic consists of those interested in health. The addicts in the latter context can see the physical aspects of their drug problems to be matters of health, *discontinuous* from the drug life. Furthermore, to be in the care of practicing professionals means that other aspects of an addict's health are more likely to be attended to.

Treatment of these drug problems by physicians and nurses in the context of general health care accords more dignity and less humiliation to addicts than they would find in a drug treatment program. Considering the extent to which health care facilities have been accused justly of dehumanization, this may be hard to believe. But by contrast, too many drug clinics treat addicts as guilty and unimportant people; frequently the staff members do not approve of addicts (a different attitude from disapproving of addiction); urine specimens are often demanded to "prove" that the addicts have not resorted to other drugs. Whereas a physician might want to examine urine specimens to determine dosage levels there would be little reason in a strictly health care context for an addict to lie.

The health care treatment of the problems can be cleanly separated from the jurisdiction of the courts over the addicts. It is current practice for courts to offer some convicted addicts the option of entering rehabilitation programs rather than prison. This invariably compromises various aspects of therapy, and, in particular, leads addicts to lie and conceal concerning their drug use when involved in methadone programs, for instance. If the health professionals' task were only stabilization, however, or the supervision of withdrawal at the request of the patient, the courts would have no interest in their role except as a prelude for further rehabilitation. The court's concern is with the psychological, economic, and social factors that lead the addict to criminal activity, not with the physical effects of drugs. Of course medical health professionals may find themselves in the position of being ordered by a court to detoxify a patient when both medical judgment and the desire of the addict point to opiate maintenance; the health professionals should resist such pressures as unprofessional.

Some people have argued that the medicalization of any aspect of drug rehabilitation is misguided except in dealing with emergencies of overdosing and withdrawal. They principally level their attacks against methadone programs. But whatever their merits against methadone programs, the attacks do not tell against the present proposal, as the following points illustrate.

Dorothy Nelkin describes a fundamental criticism of methadone programs.

> The addict's long-term association with a methadone program . . . involves him, not in terms of a limited medical program, but as a total person; he is a participant in a long rehabilitative process and necessarily an active, highly motivated, and responsible participant. Yet, the medical model that serves as the basis for the program defines the patient as ill and therefore relieved of individual responsibility, unable to manage his own problems. These assumptions are reinforced by the stereotype of addicts as childlike and irresponsible; they motivate many of the programs' precautions such as the daily requirement to urinate on demand and under observation. And they perpetuate the use of pejorative labels such as "cheating" to describe the continued use of narcotics by those unable to fully adapt to the demands of the program. The assumption of irresponsibility can strengthen the very dependence that may originally have led the patient to addiction.[4]

The problem in methadone clinics illustrated here is a confusion of medical professionalism with other functions of the staff that call for the clients to play other than the sick roles. The solution is to separate off the health care aspects of treatment, including the dispensing of methadone, into a strict health care context. With regard to the medical health professional, the addict does indeed play the sick role; this does have its own kind of responsibility, that of being serious about health and about what can be done to improve it. If the addicts also seek the other functions of a drug clinic, for instance the counselling or job placement services, they should do so according to roles in which they are not passive recipients but are reinforced in attempts toward making their own decisions about their own states. Although the staff of a medical clinic may have special expertise, the addict should not relate to the clinic as a controlled person but as someone using the expert services.

Administrators and medical health professionals working in methadone programs have been accused of being double agents, working ostensibly for the patients but also and sometimes more importantly for the government as well as for the health professions. With the increasing governmental regulation and control of methadone distribution, more and more of the physician's options have been proscribed.

Structurally, the methadone programs of today have adapted to the rigid controls established by federal and state agencies and by local groups. While these regulations have had beneficial effects in closing some bad programs, more frequently they have discouraged physicians from participating in any program. With rigid rules mandating every detail of treatment and teams of inspectors from five or more separate agencies combing the records of clinics for technical violations, the physician is made to feel as defensive as the addicts and is left with no real authority in his clinic.

He is told what addicts he is permitted to treat, the dosage limits and the permitted dose forms, the required frequency of clinic visits, what laboratory tests are mandated, the numbers and kinds of paraprofessional staff required to the licensing of the clinic, and he must justify a decision to continue treatment of any patient after an arbitrary period of time.[5]

On the policy proposed here, the health professionals would function directly and only as health professionals, not as agents of the government. This does not completely solve the problem of the double agent which exists in any therapeutic relationship; health professionals are always somewhat caught between the interests of their professions and those of their patients. But the medicalizing of certain aspects of drug rehabilitation reduces the extreme double-bind situation of drug programs to the merely universal double-bind situation of health professionals in all spheres.

Methadone programs as they ordinarily are administered demand (1) regularity, (2) abstinence from illegal drugs, and (3) respectful relations with the program staff involving at least minimal cordiality and commitment to the enterprise. Failure to comply with these norms often leads to rejection from the program, including deprivation of the maintaining drug. But should the health aspects of drug treatment be contingent on willingness and ability to obey these norms? That demand prevents some people from receiving health help and it signifies an unjust relation of domination and subjection. The more flexible norms for receiving health aid from family physicians and nurses or health clinics are preferable. Of course many general health clinics have been criticized for requiring behavior according to norms other than those in the culture of the people being served. But the problem in health clinics is less severe than in methadone programs. The critical demand for conformity in methadone programs is abstinence from other drugs; this may be appropriate for some forms of therapy, but it is morally irrelevant to health care.

A criticism often levied against methadone maintenance is that it substitutes one form of addiction for another. But exactly where does the evil lie in addiction? Any kind of addiction is a dependence that stands in the way of full personal autonomy and development, and so is bad. But some addictions are clearly better than others and some people perhaps have no chance for a non-addicted life; perhaps their personal circumstances are so bad that addiction to drugs is preferable to a naked confrontation with reality. The *moral* value of addiction is relative to circumstances.

Part of the complaint against methadone re-addiction, however, stems from the assumption that addiction is a disease entity, and that health treatment ought to aim at eliminating the disease, if possible. On what grounds can addiction be considered a disease? Surely there are health problems of managing the physical aspects of drug use—detoxifying or finding some maintenance level of opiates. But this should be viewed as medical management of a psychobiological problem, with the patient's personal interests and choices dictating what the medical solutions should be, that is, whether to detoxify, if so how, and if not, what to do instead. Addiction is a personal problem with psychobiological consequences; it may well be chosen as preferable to other problems.

Much of what has come to be regarded as drug rehabilitation can be separated off from "rehabilitation" thinking and made a health problem. But what about the causes and consequences of addiction that are so often addressed under the concept of rehabilitation?

III

The *Oxford English Dictionary* defines "rehabilitate" as "to restore by formal act of declaration (one degraded or attainted) to former privileges, rank, and possessions; to re-establish (one's good name or memory) by authoritative pronouncement. . . . To re-establish the character or reputation of (a person or thing); to clear from unfounded accusations or misrepresentations. . . . To replace in a previous state. . . . To restore to a previous condition; to set up again in a proper condition." The moral taint associated with one needing rehabilitation is clear in the first two definitions; but the sense of rehabilitation intended with reference to drug treatments is probably closer to the last two definitions, though carrying the moral connotation. The word "habilitate" means to endow with ability or capacity, or to furnish with means. In general, the growth and development of a person involves his or her habilitation. Drug addiction, among many other things, impairs the person's abilities and capacities, and deprives him or her of certain means for human existence. *Rehabilitation* would be the restoration of these. What might this mean concretely?

One clear and legitimate meaning of drug rehabilitation is the action of physicians and nurses to treat the physical matters of drug addiction, either by withdrawal or some kind of opiate maintenance (or by other means as they become available). This rehabilitates by eliminating or controlling the chemical effects of drug addiction. The chemical effects include not only physiological alterations in the blood, brain, and liver, but experiential ones of feeling, for instance, euphoria and narcosis. These experiential effects are directly related to the ingestion of opiates, and can be controlled by the health regulation of opiate use. They should not be confused with the larger psychological factors in experience that contribute to or result from drug addiction and the life it involves. Those larger psychological effects are not directly controlled in health care rehabilitation. From a health care point of view, the impairment involved in opiate addiction is that the direct physical and experiential effects of the chemicals harm the addict's life in its larger dimensions. The *definition* of harm, however, is not a health care matter. Rather it depends on the contours of the person's whole life. Health care treatment should aim at controlling the chemical effects of drug use for the sake of serving the larger interests of the addict's life.

Beyond the common physical and experiential factors of addiction, the problems of addicts can be those of anyone, particularly those in similar social situations. The young, black, ghetto addict, for instance, needs a job; but so do many young, black, ghetto non-addicts. To help addicts improve their psychological, economic, social, and personal lives, many different things may be required. Most addicts need special help. But the special help they need, other people need too: job placement, psychological counseling, perhaps a supervised residence or help in getting an apartment, a nudge toward forming social relationships through recreational activities, and a host of other things. Interestingly these are many of the same services needed by ex-mental patients, ex-convicts, the marginally retarded, and a variety of other groups.

There is no reason to group these services or human resources together under the heading of a drug treatment program. They are simply services for a variety of people who for diverse reasons may be disadvantaged with respect to them. They do not rehabilitate drug addicts but provide "habilitations" to the classes of people defined as needing those capacities.

The concept of drug rehabilitation is mischievous beyond its employment in the health care context. It misleads society, the addicts, and those who intend to help them into believing that there is a technological cure for the drug problem. This is wrong for several reasons.

First, there is no such thing as "the drug problem" beyond those aspects dealt with medically. The psychological, social, economic, and personal problems of addicts are just that: psychological, social, economic, and personal problems. Each of those dimensions of experience has its own dynamics and should be faced head on. Of course addicts' psychological problems, for instance, are affected by their having been addicted, but that does not make them drug problems. An even worse mistake would be to say that the economic problems of addicts stem chiefly from their addiction rather than from economic factors. Once an addict's addiction   nedically eliminated or controlled, the other problems should be interpreted on their own merits. In no legitimate sense is the sum of psychological, social, economic, and personal problems a syndrome of a disease for which there is a treatment called "rehabilitation."

Second, the concept of drug rehabilitation reinforces the passivity that characterizes not only addicts but most people who are in special need of human resources. It tells the addicts that someone or some institution has the answer to their problems of life and that they should accept this. Like the medical model, it encourages addicts to play the sick role and let the doctor take care of things. But unlike the medical model, drug rehabilitation beyond medical matters does not deal with sick persons. If the addicts do not take a somewhat aggressive stance toward their life, no amount of therapy, job placement, or residential supervision will help much. The concept of rehabilitation tells them that such an aggressive stance is unnecessary.

Third, the concept of rehabilitation encourages governments and other research and social agencies not to look to the basic social and cultural roots of addiction (and other social problems) and instead to search out remedies for addiction. Of course addicted people, and those who suffer extraordinarily from other social ills, should be helped by all possible means. But when the psychological and social disasters attendant upon addicts' lives are viewed as resulting from their addiction, and constitute a condition that can be cured, the society is making its peace with all the factors other than the individuals which give rise to their problem. A more radical approach is needed, and the concept of rehabilitation tends to undermine the need for this.

Fourth, the concept of rehabilitation reinforces the social view that noncriminal deviance is to be "managed." The deviants are supposed to be taken care of; their deviant condition is thought to be one that renders them objects. In conjunction with this, those who do the rehabilitating conceive themselves to be managers superior to and dominant over those to be managed, an attitude as dangerous to the managers as to the managed, and reflecting a corruption of social relations. By contrast, conceiving of human resource agencies as services to those in need reinforces the view that the needy must take advantage of opportunities. Of course, many needy people are indeed passive; this is especially true of addicts deeply involved in drugs; but are they helped by having this passivity reinforced?

Services provided to opiate addicts to help them deal with their psychological, personal, social, and economic problems should be conceived of as "pragmatic helps" to people with certain needs, needs shared in various ways by other people.

This argument should not be taken to mean that drug programs should be dismantled. Some people might believe that, if there is no "drug problem," there is no need to provide human resource services. But this conclusion does not follow. As a general principle of social thinking, no policy ought to reduce the range of possibilities offered to people in need. Society should provide as many kinds of psychological counseling and therapy, job placement, skills training, educational opportunities, residential supervision and placement, and other "human resources" as possible. Still, a basic question haunts the present thesis: will society pay for the social services needed without a target "villain" population. Does society need to believe that drug addicts are sick and/or immoral before it will provide services for them and others? Does the social willingness to help stem from a root motive of establishing the superiority of those not addicted? Whether it does in fact, the proper moral motive for social services is the inculcation of responsible life in those who may be helped.

IV

Discussion of treatment of drug addicts has focused on the implications within social policy for developing responsibility and independence in patients. Whereas this is also important in the treatment of mental patients with psychoactive drugs (principally tranquilizers), this case focuses on locating the responsibility of society.

Whether to use psychoactive drugs on mental patients who do not want them, for what purposes those drugs might be used, and who ultimately decides about their use are questions of great urgency for professionals dealing with the mentally ill. The following remarks will discuss these questions with regard to a limited class of patients, defined with reference to three conditions. First, the class consists only of those patients who are involuntarily committed to professional care, or of those for whom "leaving" professional care is not a live option. This presumes that those patients who object to the medication and could leave would leave if they felt strongly about it. Second, the class consists only of those patients who are troublesome to other people; what "troublesomeness" consists in is itself a difficult question with serious moral consequences, but it will have to be left to another time. Those patients who refuse medication but who are not troublesome constitute a separate kind of problem. Third, the patients in this class are those for whom the medication may or may not be therapeutic: it makes no difference; this qualification obviates the technical difficulty in defining whether something is therapeutic, and also the philosophic difficulty of distinguishing between drugs that are directly therapeutic and those whose custodial benefits are indirectly therapeutic on the patient or others. To sum up, the class to be considered consists of those patients for whom leaving professional care over disputes about medication is not an option, who are troublesome, and for whom the therapeutic benefit of medication is not strictly defined.

In light of the principles articulated in Section I, and reflecting the intervening discussion, it is possible immediately to draw out an elementary policy with three points for dealing with mental patients who refuse drugs that professionals want to give them. Then certain difficulties with the policy can be explored.

The first point of the policy is that patients, like drug addicts, should be encouraged in all reasonable ways to develop responsibility by taking charge of their own recovery. This means they should participate as much as possible in the interpretation of their illness, in the establishment of a therapeutic regimen, and its evaluation.

Determining when patients are capable of responding to pressures to take responsibility is a complicated matter. Surely for many patients a beginning to care consists in *relieving* them of maddening responsibilities and reassuring them that it is OK to be sick and accept help. But as they become able to accept responsibilities they should be encouraged and challenged, particularly with regard to their own welfare and those immediately around them. If this policy were practiced not only by physicians but by nurses and all the ward staff, patients might be encouraged to take responsibility themselves for monitoring their own growth in responsibility.

The second point of the policy is that where patients do not have the capacity for responsible decision making, society, through the agency of the mental health professionals, has an obligation to bring them to the responsible capacity through cures, where possible.

Suppose a patient has developed a fairly high degree of skills in deciding about his or her own treatment, and refuses a treatment that the best professional health care judgment deems necessary, or most efficient by far, for improvement. Consider, for instance, a patient who sometimes but not always hallucinates; suppose the patient refuses medications that might cause tardive dyskinesia because of greater concern about irreversible neurological problems than about transient hallucinations. Even though the professional staff may hold different values, the patient's judgment might be capable in this matter. If the patient's judgment is indeed responsible, though perhaps mistaken, then the patient's word should carry the day. Yet it would be difficult to judge that the patient were capable of responsible decision if the patient did not also have some plan for dealing with the hallucination. That is, a person capable of responsible decisions regarding mental health would need, and demonstrate, an integrated enough personality to make decisions in the light of the whole range of his or her mental health problems. Society has an obligation, according to this point of the policy, to bring patients to the capacity for responsible decision making regarding health, even if the patients do not want it. So, for instance, a severely depressed patient who refuses anti-depressant medication should be given it anyway until such time as the depression has lifted sufficiently for responsible decision making.

The third point of the policy is that where there is no therapeutic process known, and where the mental patient egregiously interferes with the safety, autonomy, or the chance for increasing responsibility in others, the interference should be restrained. Custodial restraints should be efficient according to moral criteria of efficiency, and it is an empirical question whether tranquilizers are properly efficient. Among the criteria would be effectiveness, a minimum of lasting harmful effects, a maximizing of the conditions conducive to responsible behavior, and ease of safeguarding against use for punitive rather than custodial purposes. It appears that psychoactive drugs, aversive and operant conditioning, psychosurgery, and forced seclusion each score differently on those diverse criteria. The point of the policy, however, is that patients should be efficiently restrained, even without direct therapeutic advantage, when their failure to behave responsibly in the hospital community endangers or deprives others. The justification for this point is not benefit brought to the restrained patient but responsibilities satisfied with regard to others in the community.

The first difficulty with this three-point policy is in determining what to do when conflicts arise between the points. Suppose, for instance, that in light of the first point it would be advisable to let the patient decide about a particular element of treatment and learn from the experience. But according to the second point a patient's mistaken decision might cause a serious setback in the development of responsibility, for instance the return of severe thought disorders in schizophrenia. Or suppose that from the standpoint of other people a patient should be restrained, but from the standpoint of his or her own development of responsibility, the social engagement, however painful to others, is therapeutic. All of these potential conflicts must be balanced off by trying to find the best mix in each situation. It is doubtful that there is any higher principle to appeal to that would order these three for all cases. This moves the problem to a new issue.

Who should make the decisions in these matters? One might suggest that the individual patients should make the decisions. But with regard to conflicts between choosing and therapy, patients can believe and represent themselves to be capable when they are not. With regard to conflicts between therapy and the need for custodial restraint, other people besides the individual patient have legitimate interests in the matter, and should not have their interests decided by the very one who threatens them.

The usual belief is that the physicians in charge make the decisions in cases of conflict. But physicians are often remote from the context of the decisions. For instance, it is the attending staff and perhaps other patients who engage the patient in responsible decision making hour by hour; some of them also administer and monitor the psychoactive drugs, and their environment affects the meaning which the drug has for the patient as therapeutic or merely custodial. Most forms of custodial restraint, too, are shaped by others than physicians.

So it might be said that the entire professional staff, perhaps with participation from other patients and family, should make the decision. But how is the decision to be arrived at? Majority vote is at least as insensitive to the realities of influence on the patient as physician decision making, if not more so. Physicians, nurses, and many others have both specialized expertise and individualized interests that need to be given differential weight in the decision making. No solution is offered here except to observe that the decisions *de facto* are the outcome of a group process, where the hospital group is nested in a larger society with responsibilities assigned to physicians, nurses, and others. Genuine abilities of leadership, rather than mere expertise at mere technical matters, should distinguish the weight given to individual contributions to the process. But leadership itself is defined by its own responsibilities, not by mere effectiveness, and one of the responsibilities of leadership is inserting the influence of expertise at the right time.

V

The discussion may now step back and reflect on the orientation of the remarks made so far. In asserting the great importance of personal responsibility and the obligation of society to foster it in individuals, a rationale has been provided for care of mental patients and drug addicts that differs from the customary one.

Customarily, the rationale for all medical therapeutics is that patients seek help from the health professionals; since the patients cannot cure themselves, the professionals act as the patients' agents. To protect against abuses, in many areas of health care we customarily insist upon informed consent; this means that the professional's activity is guaranteed, in principle at least, to be an extension of the patient's will. Where the patient cannot give consent, we call upon proxies who are supposed to act for the patient, not usually for the professional or the society. But this customary rationale does not work well for mental illness, and not at all for drug addiction. In the first place, in most cases the patient's will is crazy, the very thing that needs treatment; the professionals ordinarily would do harm by being extensions of that will. Furthermore, proxies ordinarily are too removed from the situation to make properly sensitive judgments and are thus at the mercy of what the professionals tell them. Finally, and most important perhaps, the rationale of the professional acting as an agent of the patient obscures both social realities and social obligations.

Instead of that rationale, the situation has been analyzed from the rationale that mental health itself is a responsibility and that society has the responsibility to foster and develop it, other things being equal. According to this rationale the professional staff acts as the agent of society, serving society's interest in making the patients more responsible.[6] This rationale does abrogate the primacy of the patients' control over the therapeutic process; but *only* on the condition that the patients are incapacitated from having responsibilities and exercising them. The rationale demands the exercise of patient control over the therapeutic process where this itself fosters the development of responsibility. Concrete freedom and responsibility are important on this rationale, whereas only their abstract shadows are important on the self-control rationale.

This social rationale for patient treatment is frankly political. It acknowledges that real power in the therapeutic-custodial situation lies in the hands of the experts and keepers, and urges that this power be subjected to constant public scrutiny and criticism. Professional staff should develop habits of self-criticism; there should be ombudsmen outside the group representing the interests of patients. Since professional staffs are agents of the society, licensing procedures and frequent reviews should be explicit, enforced, and subject to public debate. There should be more, not less, malpractice litigation; and insurance programs should be arranged so that professionals find it in their interest to testify against incompetent colleagues, giving peer review real meaning. Perhaps most important, the concrete meaning of capabilities of responsible behavior in various areas of life need to be articulated and debated, with relevant input from all sections of the public; otherwise the pet philosophy of the local professionals will be imposed on needy mental patients. This happens now, where it is not displaced by the pet philosophy of the local patient advocate. What is necessary is to make the political process of health care responsible through explicit public accountability.

Endnotes

1. Vincent P. Dole and Marie Nyswander, "Methadone Maintenance Treatment: A Ten Year Perspective," *Journal of the American Medical Association* 235, no. 1 (May 1976), pp. 2117-2119.
2. *Ibid.*
3. Avram Goldstein, Ralph Hansteen, and William Horns, "Control of Methadone Dosage by Patients," *Journal of the American Medical Association* 234, no. 7 (November 1975), pp. 734-737.
4. Dorothy Nelkin, *Methadone Maintenance: A Technological Fix* (New York: George Braziller, 1973).
5. Dole and Nyswander, "Methadone Maintenance Treatment," p. 2119.
6. For a more complete discussion of this point, see the articles on "Behavior Control" and "Drug Use, Abuse, and Dependence" by Robert Neville in the *Encyclopedia of Bioethics* (New York: Free Press, 1978).

Nursing never remains very long at the level of philosophical abstraction. The emergency nature of nursing responsibilities does not allow nurses much time for speculation. The following essay by Diane Deegan McCrann moves us quickly from the general nursing policy decisions required of nursing professionals which we have been considering in the previous two essays and confronts us with a specific case. This case, harrowing though it is, reflects precisely the moral and ethical issues that the professional nurse has to face in her practice daily. It soon becomes clear that the actual situation of nursing practice is extremely complex in that conditions exist at levels beyond the nurse's control which themselves determine significantly the type of moral response which may be made. If one implication of McCrann's essay is that a thorough reformation of the hospital's procedures is in order, then perhaps one has gained an insight into the problems facing nurses who wish to be professionals within their working situation.

13

Ethical Issues of Behavior Modification

Diane Deegan McCrann

In the following paper I wish to consider a number of ethical issues involved in the procedure known as behavior modification. My paper will present a case study and a statement of the problem presented by the particular case. After identifying pertinent clinical data and ethical issues, I shall discern ethical issues emerging from the case and offer a framework of theory for meeting these issues. I shall also consider briefly some implications of my position for public policy.

Jane Doe is a twenty-one-year-old nurse who developed a high temperature and severe abdominal pain and was admitted one morning to the surgical ward of a teaching hospital for evaluation. The admission procedure consisted of a complete history and physical examination, including a pelvic examination, by the fourth-year medical student.

That afternoon, the junior resident reviewed the student's history and physical report and decided that a second pelvic examination was necessary in order to determine whether the medical student's diagnosis of pelvic inflammatory disease was accurate. With some persuasion and explanation on the part of the junior resident, Jane agreed to a second examination. During the procedure she experienced excrutiating pain, which she found unbearable, and she demanded that the examination be stopped. The junior resident ceased the examination, expressing to Jane that he was sorry that the procedure had been so painful for her. He further explained that he was very concerned that she might have a ruptured tubal pregnancy or a ruptured appendix. For this reason he told her that it would be necessary to seek the advice and experience of the senior resident.

When the senior resident arrived in the examining room, Jane became extremely upset—crying and protesting loudly that she could not go through another pelvic examination. For thirty minutes, both physicians tried unsuccessfully to reassure her, or to gain her cooperation in a third examination. An examination of her abdomen revealed increased rigidity and rebound tenderness. Her temperature was now 104 and her pulse rate 120. Her blood pressure was 102/70. The senior resident made the assessment that Miss Doe was not only hysterical, but acutely ill, and not capable of a rational decision at this time. In order to facilitate a diagnosis and begin treatment, Jane was restrained briefly while IV Valium was administered. The pelvic examination was performed. The problem which emerges from this case is this: did the physician have the right to restrain Jane and administer IV Valium in order to examine her?

The clinical data are as follows: Jane, a twenty-one-year-old female, willingly comes to the hospital, admits herself, and seeks assistance for abdominal pain. The bureaucratic protocol at any teaching hospital consists of a history and physical by the medical student, junior resident, and so on. Health care in a teaching hospital consists of patient care *and* educational preparation of physicians.

Medical protocols for treatment are derived from years of medical experience and knowledge. These protocols are generally accepted and sanctioned by the profession and the general public. The medical model focus is one of pathology, where goals are aimed at the identification and treatment of disease entities. Evaluation of abdominal pain is a difficult differential diagnosis. History and physical data are crucial in arriving at a diagnosis. Time is a critical factor when symptoms of hemorrhage, sepsis, or peritonitis are present. In approaching a twenty-one-year-old female, the most likely differential diagnoses would include pelvic inflammatory disease, ectopic pregnancy, and appendicitis. The senior resident is faced with making a correct diagnosis through available physical findings in order to present this diagnosis to the patient and begin treatment.

Jane is a Registered Nurse who freely chooses admission into a teaching hospital for reasons not stated (confidence in system? friendships within system? works in system?). Her experience is now one of pain, fear, acute illness, and alienation from her usual role and environment. Her support systems are not known to us.

Jane is twenty-one and thus is of legal age. Her admission to the hospital is a voluntary one. The American Hospital Association "Bill of Rights" declares that "a patient must give informed consent prior to any procedure and/or treatment . . . and has the right to refuse treatment to the extent permitted by law."

From this case we can raise a number of questions that reflect on basic ethical issues. These include the following:

Does Jane have the right to refuse the examination?
Does Jane have a right to self-determination?
Does the physician have a duty to perform the examination?
Does the physician have an obligation to make a diagnosis?

Further, we can ask the basic questions arising from this case:

Is it ever justified to use coercive drug therapy to promote behavior control?

Does the right to health ever take priority over the rights to liberty, autonomy, and self-determination?

The focus of my argument, as patient advocate, emphasizes the principles of free will, human dignity, self-determination, and informed consent. My view of each individual as an autonomous being is founded in the following discussion of his or her right to a free and independent existence.

Feinberg defines rights as "valid claims which may have basis in rules governed by law or by moral principles based on convention, ideals, conscience and exercise." He defines human rights as "generically moral rights of a fundamentally important kind held equally by all human beings, unconditionally and unalterably."[1] To Feinberg, only a few human rights are absolute or universal. In this category he includes those rights which are attributed to the human state which command a higher kind of responsibility and dignity than is accorded to lower animals. Specifically, he includes the rights not to be brainwashed, not to be rendered as a docile instrument for the purposes of others, and not to be made into a domesticated animal. These universal and unalterable rights are the foundation of my argument against the use of drugs for coercive behavior control.

Throughout his writings, Veatch has consistently emphasized a commitment to individual freedom and self-determination, and the concomitant need to limit the power and authority of the medical profession. In discussing a patient's right to refuse treatment, Veatch makes the claim that an adult may refuse any treatment so long as he or she is competent, and the principal determination to be made is whether the patient is competent.[2] For Veatch, this decision rests in the courts rather than the medical profession. In this case study, the question becomes one of deciding whether Jane was intellectually capable of exercising discrimination and choice. The physician, judging her to be hysterical, defined Jane's behavior as irrational and made the decision to intervene in *her* "best interests."

Gustafson would interpret such an act as a violation of Jane's right to determine her own bodily destiny.[3] His moral assumption is that individuals have a right to refuse treatment even when in the judgment of others that treatment is in the patient's own best interest. Jane had the right to determine her own destiny.

The philosophical justification for the individual right to self-determination has been made in various ways: the right is "natural;" the capacity for self-determination is what makes humans distinctive and from this is derived both its value and its right; individual rights are conferred by God.

Are Jane's capacities to judge rationally and to act in accordance with a rational judgment impaired by her illness to the extent that she cannot properly exercise her moral right to self-determination? Did her painful experience during examinations, or her fear of another examination render her incompetent to exercise free will?

Only a highly paternalistic individual would respond *yes*.

There is a fundamental principle that encompasses free will, dignity, and self-determination. Kant spoke of it as self-rule, while Dworkin and others refer to it as autonomy.[4]

To Dworkin, autonomy consists of authenticity and independence. He recognizes each person as possessing a unique and true self, composed of unique beliefs, ideas, and actions. The greatest exercise of autonomy then is to express that nature of one's self without being subject to the will of another. To Dworkin, any method that interferes with an individual's ability to reflect on her or his motivation should not be used.

Decisions about the use of drugs to control behavior and experience are essentially choices about what is meaningful and valued in life. All drugs alter the individual's experience of life and her or his corresponding behavior. These drugs intervene directly into the internal physiological and biochemical environment. Is there not greater personal freedom when no drug is given?

The individual has the right to control her or his own behavior, and body experience, and is free to chose drug intervention if she or he desires. However, when restraints are placed on her or his behavior through drug coercion, as in the case of Jane, personal freedom has been violated. Kant, Feinberg, Gustafson, Veatch, and Dworkin would all agree that no medical reasoning or appeal to paternalism can justify drug use for behavior control. "The right of the individual to personal liberty, to self-determination to be as free as possible from the coercive power of the state remains central to our concept of the worth and dignity of man."[5]

Individuals, perceived to be normal, are given the right to make numerous choices about their lives, which by many standards may be against their self interest. They are free to lead unhealthy lives, to refuse medical treatment, to be self-destructive, and to express widely disparate views about the world. Lawyers appear comfortable safeguarding the rights of their clients with free choice left to the individual in determining his or her interests and behavior.

Why do physicians in certain circumstances fail to safeguard an individual's right to freedom? They raise questions of the nature of an individual's free will and freedom of choice under the duress of physical and mental illness. In the name of paternalism, desiring to save the patient from harming her- or himself, they "justify" coercion. "We act in the best interest of the individual and in accordance with his unconscious intent" they proclaim. The blatant and ir-responsible use of such power is a denial of the respect and dignity due to every human being.

Many physicians feel that decision making is their domain preeminently and not that of the philosopher or ethicist. They claim that the immediate experience of a situation, the persons actually involved, the suffering, and the affective states created in the physician by that experience are the most reliable indicators of what one "ought to do" in that particular situation.

Brockway explores the validity of such a claim and concludes that direct experience is not alone a sufficient safeguard against medical errors.[6] How often does it happen that a physician listens but fails to hear what another is saying, or that the physician infers from the patient's choices or actions the presence of certain interests or beliefs, which are actually not present at all.

Direct or immediate experience is not necessary in order to come to know the information one needs to know in making a moral judgment, nor is it any guarantee that the information one gets is not mistaken. The claim that the physician's first-hand experience of the situation places him or her in a privileged position relative to those who do not have such first-hand experience does not succeed. Such a claim rests more on a defense of territory than on moral grounds.

An acute illness alone does not create a justifiable basis for forced administration of psychoactive drugs to anyone who refuses to take them voluntarily. In this case study, Jane explicitly expressed a desire *not* to have a third pelvic examination. Such a statement assumes a rejection of any drug which would negate her willful behavior to prevent such an examination from taking place. It appears that trust has no significant value in the relationship between Jane and the senior resident.

It is common belief that the relationship between a patient and physician is dependent upon trust. Wherein does the trust lie, and who justifies it? For Freedman, the belief that the physician has the knowledge necessary to treat illness is not enough; trust in physicians who serve in institutions is notoriously lacking, although their knowledge is not in question. Rather, this trust is predicated upon a firm belief that the physician is acting solely and steadfastly in the patient's own interests.

A model of medical care according to Freedman lists three interrelated implications:

1. The patient decides when and if he ought to seek medical care and advice, and once given, has the choice of whether to accept treatment or not.
2. Assuming the patient decides to remain under medical care, the patient becomes a partner in preserving and or restoring his health. (The moral implication is that the MD is no longer solely responsible for the medical intervention performed on the patient.)
3. The patient defines health and illness for himself.[7]

This contemporary model preserves autonomy and gives the responsibility and freedom of choice to each individual. The physician is responsible for his or her own actions; the patient for his or hers.

A deontological approach to ethical decisions, in which the rightness of the act is independent of any consequence of that act, appears to be most consistent with my argument in this case. My concern is whether an act will conform with moral principles or laws or will violate them. The problem is whether it is ethical for the senior resident to have given IV Valium in order to change Jane's behavior and facilitate an examination.

In review, we have a situation in which the alternatives available to the senior resident were to give IV Valium or not to do so. We find that it is not consistent with the general principles and duties pertaining to his profession for him to do so. The general principles include those relating to the patient's autonomy, rights of informed consent, self-determination, free will, and the issues of beneficence and non-maleficence. The physician's duties pertaining here are to do no harm, to preserve human dignity, to preserve privacy, to preserve autonomy, and to maintain trust in the physician–patient relationship.

Under no circumstances was the physician justified in the use of IV Valium to facilitate an examination of Jane. It is my belief that alternatives such as offering Jane a choice in the use of medication or an opportunity to discuss her concerns with a nurse and/or family member would have exhibited a more humanistic approach to resolving the conflict. In the hierarchy of beneficence, according to Frankenna, the command to do no harm always takes precedence over preventing or removing harm, or even promoting good. A harmful act was committed against Jane by the physician's use of IV Valium. Such a drug rendered Jane helpless and vulnerable to the will of the physician and the institution. Any free expression of Jane's autonomy was quickly extinguished. Clearly other alternatives, if pursued, would have maintained Jane's rights and fulfilled the physician's obligations.

Finally, only a highly paternalistic society would tolerate the intrusions upon autonomy and privacy that flow from a coercive act such as the one I have just discussed.

If public policy reflected my decision that the coercive use of drugs for behavior control is never justified, the following assumptions might be made:

Isolated irrational behaviors inconsistent with an individual's usual personhood might threaten the physical and mental integrity of that individual.

An actual loss of autonomy secondary to mental or physical illness might not be restored because drug use would be prevented.

Violations of personal freedom and rational expressions of autonomy would not occur.

Institutions and individual professionals prone to paternalistic behavior would not have the opportunity to "misinterpret" an individual's unconscious wishes.

Alternatives to drug use might include improved communication and involvement of family and friends to reduce the alienation of an individual.

Endnotes

1. J. Feinberg, *Social Philosophy*. (Englewood Cliffs, New Jersey: Prentice-Hall, 1973).
2. R. Veatch, "Drugs and Competing Drug Ethics," *Hastings Center Report*, 1972, pp. 68–80.
3. J. Gustafson, "'Ain't Nobody Goin Cut on My Head!'" *Hastings Center Report*, February 1975, pp. 49–51.
4. G. Dworkin, "Autonomy and Behavior Control," *Hastings Center Report*, February 1976, pp. 23–29.
5. J. Himmelstein, "The Right to Refuse Psychoactive Drugs," *Hastings Center Report*, June 1973, pp. 8–11.
6. G. Brockway, "The Physician's Appeal to Firsthand Experience," *Hastings Center Report*, April 1976, pp. 9–11.
7. B. Freedman, "The Case for Medical Care, Inefficient or Not," *Hastings Center Report*, April 1977, pp. 31–39.

Bibliography

Beauchamp, T. and Walters, L. *Contemporary Issues in Bioethics*. Encino, Calif.: Dickenson Publishing Co., 1978.

Brockway, G. "The Physician's Appeal to Firsthand Experience," *Hastings Center Report*, April 1976, 9–11.

Dworkin, G. "Autonomy and Behavior Control," *Hastings Center Report*, February 1976, 23–29.

Feinberg, J. *Social Philosophy*. Englewood Cliffs, N. J.: Prentice Hall, Inc., 1973.

Freedman, B. "The Case for Medical Care, Inefficient or Not," *Hastings Center Report*, April 1977, 31–39.

Gustafson, J. "Ain't Nobody Goin Cut on My Head!" *Hastings Center Report*, February 1975, 49–51.

Himmelstein, J. "The Right to Refuse Psychoactive Drugs," *Hastings Center Report*, June 1973, 8–11.

Jonas, H. "The Right to Die," *Hastings Center Report*, August 1978, 31–36.

Klerman, G. "Behavior Control and the Limits of Reform," *Hastings Center Report*, August 1975, 40–45.

Klerman, G. "Psychotropic Drugs as Therapeutic Agents," *Hastings Center Report*, 1974, 87–94.

Macklin, R. "Moral Concerns and Appeals to Rights and Duties," *Hastings Center Report*, October 1976, 31–38.

Reich, W. "The Physician's Duty to Preserve Life," *Hastings Center Report*, April 1975, 14–15.

Veatch, R. "Drugs and Competing Drug Ethics," *Hastings Center Report*, 1972, 68–80.

One of the most intriguing of ancient as well as modern medical practices is that of administering to patients materials which have no medical or therapeutic values whatsoever. To the unreflective individual such a practice seems not to present much of a problem. After all, what harm is done if a patient thinks she or he is getting something of value when she or he is not? Maybe the patient will even get better due to her or his own psychological satisfaction at having been given something that she or he feels will be of assistance. What harm? Only the harm, as Patricia O'Neil makes quite clear, of deception, the harm of making the nurse an accomplice of deception, and only the harm of violating both the codes of honesty and simple truth-telling applicable to every member of society—medical doctors included. O'Neil's study shows that placebo administration has a colorful history within medical practice. She also reviews a considerable literature on the subject and shows that the matter of administration of placebos is not a simple black-and-white issue. Much good can come from placebo administration. The question is this: what shall the professional nurse's responsibility be in this instance?

14

Placebo Administration: An Ethical Issue

Patricia A. O'Neil

In this paper I wish to discuss the ethical and legal implications of employing placebos as drug therapy. Among issues to be considered will be those of deception, truth-telling, informed consent, and the doctor–patient, nurse–patient relationship. These ethical considerations will be recognized in terms of individual autonomy, free will, and the individual's right to self-determination. The pros and cons of placebo therapy will be explored, alternatives will be given and analyzed. The ultimate goal is to arrive at a nursing proposal regarding the use of placebos in medical and nursing practice.

> When a man's life has become bound up with the analytic technique, he finds himself at a loss altogether for the lies and the guile which are otherwise so indispensable to a physician, and if for once with the best intentions he attempts to use them, he is likely to betray himself. Since we demand strict truthfulness from our patients, we jeopardize our whole authority if we let ourselves be caught by them in a departure from the truth.
>
> Sigmund Freud
> Collected Papers, II

Let us begin by defining our terms. A placebo is any therapeutic procedure (or that component of any therapeutic procedure) that is given deliberately to have an effect, or unknowingly has an effect, on a patient, symptom, syndrome, or disease but that is objectively without specific physiological activity for the condition being treated. The therapeutic procedure may be given with or without conscious knowledge that the procedure is a placebo, may be an active (noninert) or non-active (inert) procedure, and includes, therefore, all medical procedures no matter how specific: oral and parenteral medication, topical preparations, inhalents, and mechanical, surgical, and psycho-therapeutic procedures.[1]

A "pure" placebo is an inert substance, lactose or sugar tablet, distilled water or saline injection, which is physiologically, biologically, and organically inactive.[2] An "impure" or "adulterated" placebo contains some active ingredient, but one that has no effect on the patient's illness; the active substance may be inappropriate to the disease entity or in a subtherapeutic dose.[3]

The "placebo effect" is the psychological, physiological, or psychophysiological effect of any medication or procedure given with therapeutic intent, which is independent of, or minimally related to, the pharmacologic effects of the procedure, and which operates through a psychological mechanism.[4]

A lie is an intentionally deceptive message that is stated.[5] Deception is the communication of messages meant to mislead and meant to make others believe what one him- or herself does not believe; this can be accomplished through gestures, disguise, by means of action or inaction, even through silence.[6]

The use of placebos coupled with the placebo effect can be traced back to the origins of humanity. It is believed by some that the placebo and its effect is the fundamental link between ancient and modern medical practice.

Documentation of therapy which appears today to have had placebic effect dates back as far as 1500 B.C. in ancient Egypt. There, according to the Ebers Papyrus, patients were often treated with medications such as "lizard's blood, crocodile dung, the teeth of swine, the hoof of an ass, putrid meat and fly specs." In the seventh century A.D., Paul of Aegina detailed uses of blood from a number of animal species to treat conditions as diverse as dropsy, poor visual acuity, dyspnea, kidney stones, epilepsy, and cerebral hemorrhages. The seventeenth century *London Pharmacopeia* recommended worms, dried viper, oil of frog sperm, human perspiration, spider's webs, and usnea-moss, material scraped from the skull of a hanged criminal, to treat a multitude of conditions.[7] In the 1800s, bleeding was a fashionable therapy to cure almost any ailment. Leeches provided a popular method to facilitate this practice. In 1827 alone, 33,000,000 leeches were imported into France because domestic supplies were exhausted.[8]

Consider the following treatment followed by physicians treating King Charles II:

A pint of blood was extracted from his right arm, and a half pint from his left shoulder, followed by an emetic, two physics, and an enema comprising fifteen substances; the royal head was then shaved and a blister raised; then a sneezing powder, more emetics, and bleeding, soothing potions, a plaster of pitch and pigeon dung on his feet, potions containing ten different substances, chiefly herbs, finally drops of extract of human skull and the application of bezoar stone; after which his majesty died.[9]

Despite the ridiculous, often harmful methods of treatment, the physician continued to be a revered and respected, highly prestigious member of society. It can be safely concluded that the widespread acceptance of past medical practice was based primarily on placebo effect. It was not until the seventeenth century, when Syndeham isolated quinine from cinchoma bark as a treatment for fever of malarial origin, that scientific medicine began to emerge. Early medicine owes its success undoubtedly to the doctor–patient relationship, with its basis of trust, and the realization of the powerful therapeutic qualities of the doctor her- or himself. Success was also founded in fate; the fate of spontaneous recoveries that occurred despite and coincidentally with the placebo. The elements of enthusiasm, suggestibility, trust, and desire to improve health may also have been instrumental in effecting a cure.[10] The same reasons can apply to the effectiveness and widespread use of placebo therapy today, with one major difference. The folk doctors of the past, in their ignorance and desire to treat effectively, prescribed the bizarre medicines mentioned above. Today, medical technology and scientific research has enabled people to rationally investigate and discover medications specific to certain disease entities, yet placebo therapy flourishes. Let us examine the current practice of placebo therapy.

One author makes the astute observation that 60 to 80 percent of the case load carried by the general practitioner constitutes illnesses defined as functional, such as hypochondriasis, psychophysiological disturbances, and most emotional disorders; all, he contends, treatable by placebo therapy.[11] In Great Britain, a conservative estimate concludes that one-third of all health service prescriptions fall into the placebo category.[12]

The literature abounds with shady testimony of the widespread use of placebos. Most of the statements consider placebo therapy crucial to effective medicine and justify its use with paternalistic rationale and strong adherence to Plato's theory in the *Republic*,". . . a lie is useful only as a medicine to men, confined to physicians."[13]

Medicine today is not just caring for and about one's patients; it is big business. The more patients seen, the more the financial gratification realized. As Dr. J. candidly states:

I should say that 90% of my consultations end in a prescription. Most of this is placebo therapy, a lot of it for neurotic conditions. They seem to see that something is being done for them if you write out a "script." A person will come in here and say: "I feel terrible, doctor! Can I have a tonic?" Well, you can either go into all the ramifications and find out why they are depressed, which may take you two hours, or you can simply say that you would be prepared to listen to them but you haven't the time. You are offering them this bottle of medicine instead. You give them a cheap tonic that is in the standard book.[14]

Dr. J. illustrates how the routine prescription of a placebo can forestall lengthy discussion in the office. He also suggests it is an economical means of demonstrating his concern for the patient's well-being.

Most physicians, though probably similar to Dr. J., are less comfortable with their use of placebos, yet placebos continue to be a major treatment modality of many doctors. In a study done by Dr. Charles Hofling in 1955, when physicians were asked how often they used placebos in their practice three times as many doctors questioned were of the belief, perhaps with a certain degree of selfdeception, that they used placebos less frequently than was average practice. Basically, the average physician preferred to think of her- or himself as needing to resort to placebos less frequently than colleagues. Dr. Hofling also ascertained that placebos were often employed in situations where the physician's knowledge was inadequate to the problem. Therefore, the use of placebos and their subsequent discussion can represent a threat to the physician's self-esteem.[15] Dr. Hofling seems to imply that associated with this threat to self-esteem that is experienced by doctors who prescribe placebos is a lack of candor and truthfulness regarding the prevalence of the actual use of placebos.

There are certainly other indications for placebo use as determined by the medical profession.

Dr. Beecher sees utilization of placebos beneficial as a psychological instrument in the therapy of certain ailments originating in mental illness; placebos are a resource for the harrassed MD in dealing with a neurotic patient; they can also be used to determine the true effects of drugs apart from suggestion in experimental work; and lastly, Dr. Beecher cites the placebo as a valuable device for eliminating bias in experimentation, not only on the part of the subject but also when used as an unknown by the observer.[16] Others are more definitive in their proposed uses: in research with informed consent; to wean patients off narcotics and sedatives; in the terminally ill, as helpful in lessening narcotic-induced side effects like respiratory depression. Placebo administration is advocated as a substitute for a conglomerate of useless drugs that a patient may be taking to aid in problem identification; as a form of psychotherapy; and, lastly, placebos merit use to calm hospitalized patients or those who are impatient regarding a diagnosis forcing the MD to prescribe something "in the meantime," "as most patients do not understand that diagnosis must precede intelligent treatment."[17]

Once it has been decided to employ a placebo as treatment, the process begins to become more complex. Apparently, a definite method of deceit must be initiated. A good place to begin is with the actual writing of the prescription. The well-known illegibility of the prescription assures concealment from the patient of the actual medication prescribed. If one is at all able to decipher the scrawling, it is usually in Latin and therefore frequently just as irrelevant.

To insure that the patient does not ask the pharmacist to serve as interpreter, the physician is advised against ordering such commonly known ingredients as milk sugar or saline. There are a multitude of offensive tasting and vividly colored potions which are not only impressive in physical qualities but also possess names guaranteed to make any doubting Thomas a firm believer. Names such as "ammoniated tincture of valerian can be safely revealed to the patient without upsetting the psychological applecart."[18] Another important consideration that must not be overlooked is that a significant number of prescriptions are now paid for by third-party carriers. These carriers will not pay for inert placebos, forcing the pharmacist to notify recipients that their prescription is non-specific to their ailment. Consequently, many patients feel duped and victimized by deceitful practice. The web only becomes more intricate as it is suggested that to avoid the aforementioned situation the physician has two choices. First, she or he can notify the pharmacist of the circumstances and enlist her or his support in the deception, or she or he can dispense the placebos from her or his office and avoid any confrontation with an uncooperative pharmacist or unobliging third-party carrier.[19]

The charade continues as documentation has been compiled to indicate what the most effective placebo should resemble. Color is an important consideration, as it suggests more specificity than a transparent capsule or pill. Tasteless remedies are basically ineffective and unimpressive as people tend to associate vile tasting preparations with a cure. Overly large pills or very tiny ones are more conducive to relief than the average aspirin-size tablet, as they imply potency. Naturally, injections warrant more relief than pills, presumably related to the presence of a doctor or a nurse who administers the shot. All of these guidelines, while perfecting deceit, add psychotherapeutic punch![20]

Why placebos work has opened many avenues of speculation. First and foremost, success is credited to the doctor–patient relationship, and it is claimed that any health care system that minimizes or fragments the doctor-patient relationship will also lessen the efficiency of the placebo effect.[21] Studies have documented that the more conviction the doctor can muster in her or his deception, the more effective the placebo will be.[22] It is believed that the placebo effect starts long before the first pill is taken. It begins with the initial encounter between the doctor and patient. If the patient does not sense comfort and understanding from this first meeting, the likelihood of the positive placebo response is diminished.[23] Other indicators of a positive or successful response depend on the patient's and the MD's expectation of relief. The patients' confidence in the prescribed therapy, combined with their previous experience with medications (assuming it is positive), and the enthusiasm with which the placebo is given complement the patients' positive response.[24]

Physicians with faith in the efficiency of their treatment, who can allow that enthusiasm to be projected to their patients, along with strong expectations of specific side effects and who themselves are confident and attentive, can most often elicit a positive placebo response from their patients.[25] It is evident that placebos derive their power from the vast potential of the emotional relationship between the omnipotent doctor and the needs of the patient. It seems as if the patient places her or his trust in the physician only to be dealt a dirty trick by the MD who is playing the role of a manipulative puppeteer, programming and evoking conditioned responses from an unsuspecting patient population, all under the guise of benevolent deception. The relationship that is developed and based on trust is maintained on a false pretense. The perpetuation and indoctrination of the traditional physician–patient relationship has allowed this passivity of the patient to nurture, and placebo therapy to continue unchallenged.

The effectiveness of placebo therapy has its inherent value in the fact that the patient is kept in the dark and uninformed to maximize her or his suggestibility. If informed consent were secured with placebo therapy, then, undoubtedly, the rate of success would be lessened.

Veatch outlines three models of the doctor–patient relationship:

1. *Engineering Model:* The doctor acts as a scientist dealing only in facts; values do not enter into the decision making process. The patient is presented the cold hard facts and can decide on treatment.
2. *Priestly Model:* Paternalism is the outstanding feature of the physician in this model. The doctor makes all moral and medical decisions in this model because "he knows best."[26]
3. *Contractual Model:* This model represents a non-legalistic statement of general obligations and benefits to both parties, with a shared decision making responsibility.[27]

Brody feels we are progressing toward this last model in health care today. Once the Contractual Model is realized, informed consent in a truer sense should follow. The mutual consent that the Contractual Model implies gives the contract its essence. The consent implies an offer and acceptance. Conditions of mutual consent suggest "that it must be an external manifestation of a free internal act of the will. It must be externally manifested because a contract is between two persons and supposes communication between them. It must be internally given by a free act because a contract is a human act requiring an act of the will consequent on knowledge. Freedom of consent may be nullified by error or fear."[28]

The trend for consumer awareness and mutual participation is clearly becoming equalized in other relationships such as landlord–tenant, police–suspect, and employer–employee. The doctor–patient relationship, although slow in catching on, is now becoming more bilateral rather than unilateral. It is speculated the reason is associated with spiraling inflationary medical costs, with patients therefore demanding a larger voice in decision making pertinent to health issues. This consumer demand is dependent on accurate and adequate information from those who hold the key, the physicians.[29] Many surmise placebos are becoming "victims of consumerism." With the impetus for informed consent and patient participation in the decision making process, there will be a demise of the paternalistic physician with a rise in consumerism. Subsequently, placebos will suffer therapeutically and those who advocate placebo therapy conclude that consumerism, while negating the effectiveness of placebos, has paid a high price for its victory.[30]

When physicians are asked to substantiate and justify their seemingly flagrant use of placebos, the overwhelming response is that the patient demands it.[31] Comaroff, while studying this concept of patient demand for treatment, found one MD who believes that patients benefit from the ritual of being treated as ill. Comaroff concludes that this belief justifies the use of pseudo-scientific techniques that furnish the physician with a strategy for dealing with trivial illness in a rapid and efficient way. He found that doctors have difficulty in coming to terms with clinical action which does not include the use of drugs. He ascertains that the physician feels compelled to prescribe even a placebo to reassure her- or himself as much as the patient that she or he is offering tangible treatment.[32] The obligation to prescribe is fostered by physicians who require a concrete display to communicate therapeutic intent and attempt to cure. This, the physician justifies, reassures the patient that something is being done for him or her and that someone cares.

Medication has always seemed to be vital to humans. Sir William Osler felt that a desire to take medicine was the simple, most outstanding difference between people and animals. It is supposed that whatever relief was first obtained from people's first indulgence in medicine was due to the placebo effect.[33] Despite this favorable claim to fame, in November 1972, Gary Yingling of the Federal Drug Administration, along with members of the government, drug industry, and academia congregated at the Smithsonian Institution to discuss the placebo effect. The pressing question was, how could the F.D.A. best serve the public, by taking inert, patent medicines off the market, or by leaving well enough alone? They concluded that since placebos remain a real and important means of subjective relief for a large percentage of the population, prohibiting their use might have serious ramifications. The committee conceded that these modern day cure-alls will be around for many years to come. The style of advertising may change, names and ingredients of preparations may change, but the never-ending demand for something to swallow to correlate with symptom relief will always be present. It is this necessity that will cost us, as consumers, billions of dollars per year.[34] Dr. Hoff, a German physician, in his address to the Conference of German Physicians in Mannheim, 1963, called for stricter controls with drug advertising. It is his belief that consumer dependence on medication is directly related to the social impact of advertising and, consequently, we all know and expect chemical cures for all ailments. "One cannot buy health in a chemist's shop," declares Dr. Hoff. A mutual effort of physician and patient working collaboratively with each party accepting responsibility for itself is the avenue to palliation. Hippocrates wisely professed, "the patient must be alongside the physician in the fight against his illness."[35]

One would assume that all aspects of the use of a practice that enjoys such wide popularity as placebo therapy would be sufficiently documented in the literature. The endeavor to uncover the legal or ethical aspects of placebo therapy leaves one frustrated and without any substantial information.

In 1974, Sissela Bok discovered, while surveying medical textbooks, that many of them provided little analysis of placebo treatment. She sampled nineteen popular current textbooks in medicine, pediatrics, surgery, anesthesia, obstetrics, and gynecology and found only three even mentioned placebos. She was also disheartened to find that none of them chose to deal with the ethical, moral, or legal dilemmas placebos present.[36] In 1975, Dr. Thomas Silber requested a medline search on placebos. He secured 1,500 articles but only eighteen of these publications even recognized an ethical issue regarding placebo therapy. He acknowledges "an incongruity between the richness of the pharmacologic, therapeutic, psychiatric, and research literature on this subject in general and the scant attention paid to the moral issues involved."[37]

The legal issue of informed consent in light of placebo therapy will now be addressed, followed by moral analysis of the perplexities inherent in placebo use, concluding with a nursing proposal regarding the practice and use of placebo therapy.

> If, like truth, the lie had but one face, we would be on better terms. For we would accept as certain the opposite of what the liar would say. But the reverse of truth has a hundred thousand faces and an infinite field.
>
> Montaigne, Essays

Legally, the doctrine of informed consent implies a sharing of decision making power between the doctor and the patient.[38] Prior to 1960, the physician basically informed the patient that a procedure was to be done, then did it, often without obtaining consent. It was a common conception that when a patient placed her- or himself in the hands of the physician for care, the act implied consent to the MD to carry out all necessary and acceptable means to relieve or cure.[39]

Historically, the first case dealing with informed consent arose in the late eighteenth century, *Slater v. Baker and Stapleton*. Retribution was aimed at physicians who did not follow customary, professional standards of practice. In 1916, Justice Cardozo in *Schloendorff v. Society of New York Hospital* said, ". . . every human being has a right to determine what shall be done with his body."[40] Cases of informed consent seemed to drop off for a few decades but became very popular in the late 1950s and 1960s. Two monumental state supreme court rulings dealing with informed consent occurred in 1960 in the cases of *Natanson v. Kline* in Kansas, and *Mitchell v. Robinson* in Missouri. It was decided in each case, though consent had been given in both cases, by the court's ruling that ". . . the patient's consent was insufficient to shield the doctor's liability for untoward consequences of treatment even though the physicians were not negligent in performance of procedures." Consents were judged invalid because the MDs had not informed the patients generally of possible serious side effects.[41]

The valid giving of consent required that an individual be of sufficient mentality to make an intelligent choice to do something proposed by another. The rule of thumb seems to indicate "reasonableness" as the criterion.[42] Naturally the next question one must presuppose is, "who is a reasonable and responsible person?" There are some who feel the "reasonable person" is "a mythical creature of law, who has never been seen by the light of day but acts as a standard by which courts measure the conduct of all other persons and find it to be proper or improper."[43] The frustration of definition rests with the abstractness of the term. It changes with every case and changes as society changes. It merely implies what is currently accepted as reasonable; new definitions dynamically evolve with every case. For purposes of explanation, "a reasonable person" for the time being will consist of an individual of normal intelligence who makes prudence a guide to conduct where conduct is guided by ordinary conduct of human affairs.[44] The battle continues as courts attempt to determine just how much information physicians are compelled to deliver to a "reasonable person."

In 1972, courts in California (*Cobbs v. Grant*), and Washington, D.C. (*Cantebury v. Spence*), tried to define this amount. Decisions in these two cases solidly affirmed the patient's rights to self-determination regarding collateral risk (doctor–patient). Based on these two decisions, it was extended that physicians are bound to "reasonable disclosure."[45] Once again, that nondescript term emerges from the halls of justice. The present principle of informed consent holds that physicians must disclose all information relevant to a proposed therapy that a reasonable person would need to make an intelligent decision. Eighteen states since 1975 have enacted legislation that deals with the issue of informed consent. Regrettably, much of the legislation is an exercise in semantics. Most lawmakers who have become superficially acquainted with the issue emphasize disclosure on the part of the doctor but tend to ignore the issue of patient understanding of the disclosure, which is crucial to obtain a valid informed consent.[46] The publicity of consumer awareness in the health field led to the development by the American Hospital Association, in 1972, of the Patient's Bill of Rights. This statement clearly defines the patient as being justifiably deserving of all information to make an informed decision about his or her care. Despite this sincere attempt to distribute the power, so to speak, between physician and patient, many conclude that the Bill of Rights for patients is vague and non-specific; one source likens it to the fox telling the chickens what their rights are![47] A vast majority of medical professionals today regard informed consent as a legal obstruction to practice. They view informed consent as a formality, a slip of paper to be signed to release them from liability. Medicine beware . . . the signature on the form is not a guarantee against legal repercussions. If a patient can convince the court she or he did not read the form, or was under duress, or was not informed, the informed consent application will not be legally binding to the physician's benefit. In a justifiable case, the burden of proof rests with the hospital or the physician.[48]

The Declaration of Helsinki, adopted in 1964, was a statement defining informed consent. It was revised in 1975 with assistance from the Department of Health, Education, and Welfare. The Declaration provides for:

1. explanation of proposed treatment,
2. explanation of inherent risks and benefits,
3. alternatives to proposed treatments,
4. adequate time for patient questions,
5. option to withdraw at any time,
6. freedom from coercion, unfair persuasions, and inducements for informed consent.

It is evident that placebo therapy runs counter to many, if not all, of the ideals of informed consent. It stands to reason that the more a patient's rights are impinged upon, the more the proposed practice that is restricting these rights becomes an ethical issue.

Margaret Mead, in her opening statement at the American Academy of Arts and Sciences Conference on Human Experimentation in 1968, made the following remarks, which certainly have merit and correlations to placebo therapy:

> There is a responsibility to the subjects that they not be exposed to ridicule, legal sanctions or danger without their informed concurrence. The more powerless the subject is per se, the more the question of ethics and power is raised. It is assumed trust will follow status, therefore more precautions must be taken to see that trust is not abused. Any careless or reckless downgrading of the status of human experimentation, any denigration of human rights, any exposure to unethical procedures or submission to lying or deceit arouse fear and destroy trust.

Trust, or lack of it, seems to emerge as the key to a deceptive practice like placebo therapy. Many advocate placebo use in terms of cost-benefit analysis. The benefit the patient receives as a result of the benevolent deception justifies, according to prescribers, the use of placebos. All advocates quickly admit, though, that their greatest and primary concern is that they will be caught, a valid fear at that. While placebo effects depend essentially on deception, if indiscriminate, wide-spread use of placebos continues, eventually the word will get out and the efficacy of placebos will fade, as will trust in the medical world.[49]

R. C. Cabot, in 1909, profoundly summarized the truth and deception in medicine associated with placebos:

> The majority of placebos are given because we believe the patient has learned to expect medicine for every symptom, and without it he simply won't get well. True, but who taught him to expect a medicine for every symptom? He was not born with that expectation . . . it is we, the physicians who are responsible for perpetuating false ideas about disease and its cure . . . with every placebo that we give, we do our part in perpetuating error, and a harmful error at that.[50]

A utilitarian can rationalize benefits of some lies as necessary protocol to avoid harm. For utilitarians, a lie is more or less justifiable depending on its consequences. The moral choice is weighed and some lies are deemed more or less serious than others. In making a judgment on a lie, the degree of severity is directly related to the amount of happiness or harm the lie will entail. The problem becomes more perplexing when the lie is more complex. It is difficult enough to make assessments of utility that affect one person, keeping in mind the numerous consequences and alternatives. But to make judgment on several persons can be nearly impossible.[51]

A study done at the University of California, San Francisco, by Levine, Gordon, and Fields, has hypothesized a new dimension as to the effectiveness of placebo therapy. They propose that endomorphin activity accounts for placebo analgesia. Cortical activity stimulates endomorphins, an opium-like substance within the human body. With validation and testing, should this theory hold true, the inert placebo would have physiological importance though primarily triggered by a psychological response.[52] Placebo effect could be rationally explained with the validity of this hypothesis, but until it is proven fact, this author cannot justify placebo therapy.

By acknowledging and accepting Kant's Categorical Imperative that man is to be regarded as "an end in himself," hence no one should ever be treated merely as a means to desire-determined ends, this author will argue against placebo therapy from a deontological viewpoint. It will be illustrated that an individual is not treated as an end in her- or himself and her or his rights of individuality, freedom, dignity, self-respect, autonomy, and justice are negated with placebo therapy.

In determining an ethical stand, a model depicted by Howard Brody was utilized:

Problem Perception

The ethics of administering placebos as drug therapy

List Alternatives

1. To give placebos and not to disclose the fact
2. To not give placebos, therefore no explanation

Make a Choice; Frame an Ethical Statement

It is unethical and against an individual's rights of autonomy, freedom, dignity, self-respect and justice to administer placebos with therapeutic intent.

List Consequences of Each Alternative

To Give a Placebo

1. Patient will be satisfied with action.
2. Belief perpetuated that there is a pill for every ailment; patients will come to expect it.
3. Patient will lose confidence and trust if he finds out later it was a placebo.
4. Patient may develop side effects despite the fact it is a placebo.[53]
5. You will be personally dissatisfied by having abandoned moral principles.
6. Patient will have to pay for placebo.
7. You reinforce the erroneous notion about the proper use of drugs.

To Not Give a Placebo

1. Patient may be dissatisfied with no prescription.
2. Personal satisfaction for following own moral principles.
3. Patient may seek other medical intervention for a prescription; consequently the patient is lost.
4. No chance of side effects with no medication.
5. Patient saved price of placebo.
6. Reputation in community may suffer if patient publicly complains.
7. After explaining why you will not prescribe a drug, contribution has been made to increase patient awareness and education regarding the correct use of drugs.
8. By being honest with patient, may actually help patient and avoid costly psychiatric intervention at a later date.

The next step in Brody's model is to scan a list of personal values:

1. That every person be treated as an end in her- or himself, with rights of autonomy, freedom, dignity, self-respect, and justice respected.
2. Truth-telling.
3. Advocacy of consumer participation and awareness in health issues.
4. Therapeutic conservatism.

5. To be respected by patients.
6. To be liked by patients.

After one's personal values are determined, one must ask oneself, "would I be satisfied to have this action taken upon me?" Consequences are not regarded relative to the values defined. It is here that value conflicts are sifted and significant consequences are delineated with the higher level values. Clearly shown is that more values are preserved and consequences that appeal to higher values are consistent with not administering placebos; therefore the ethical statement made at the onset of this model is valid, based on Kant's Categorical Imperative. It is only reasonable to arrive at a conclusion that does not sanction placebo use and the deception inherent in the practice of such an intervention.

A deontological framework dictates that there are rules or moral principles of action which have moral validity independent of consequences of individual actions, and that one must act in accordance with these rules or principles. What is "right" is sometimes independent of what is "good," but an obligation exists to do what is "right" even when the "good" is not served by it. In the case illustrated, not giving the placebic remedy may cause the patient to be unhappy; he or she may seek other medical help and one's reputation may suffer in the community. Although none of these consequences can be termed "good," it is one's duty to respect individual autonomy and, therefore, not use placebos.

There are many false statements that are not intentionally deceptive. In medicine, an erroneous statement believed to be true is not deception. The guilt rests with the physician who knowingly and intentionally prescribes a placebo and benevolently rationalizes her or his deception. Intentional deception takes place when there is a flow of information between at least two individuals such that the information is believed by the transmitter to be misleading to the receiver and is intended to mislead. Such deception may be verbal, which constitutes a lie; or it can be nonverbal, communicated by gestures, false visual cues, or even silence.[54] "Uttering a falsehood is always deceptive. Omitting to provide information, on the other hand, is deceptive only where one person is silent, knowing that another will draw false inference from that silence."[55]

Lying is also contradictory to Natural Law. It is an abuse of natural ability that destroys speech, and its primary and essential end—to speak the truth. Lying is not a mere use of speech for a secondary end, leaving the primary end intact. While lying may bring about some extrinsic good, it does it by an evil means and at the expense of an intrinsic good and of an end in itself, trust and autonomy.[56] The paternalistic attitude of many physicians overlooks the age-old premise that all people are created equal. When obstruction of this equality occurs, as with paternalistic deception, an individual's rights have been threatened and freedom comprised.[57] To meddle with another's rights, thus making her or his life difficult, especially when we would not accept the same treatment ourselves, constitutes an injustice.

The paternalistic freedom behind which so many health professionals hide causes more harm and distrust than it intends. Paternalism can be regarded as the use of coercion to achieve a good that is not recognized as such by those individuals for whom the good is intended.[58] The presence of paternalism destroys any pretension of informed consent or individual freedom. The responsibility to prevent the perpetration of such a relationship lies equally with the physician, the patient, and society. The patient is responsible for exercising her or his right of autonomy, while the physician and the society are obliged to prevent encroachment on that right.[59]

Sissela Bok, in her article, "The Ethics of Giving Placebos," quotes Melvin Levine, who colorfully depicts the use (or abuse) of truth in medicine:

> . . . the medical profession has practiced as if truth is, in fact, a kind of therapeutic instrument that can be altered and given in smaller doses or not used at all when deemed detrimental to the patient . . . many M.D.'s have utilized truth distortion as a kind of anesthetic to promote comfort and ease treatment.[60]

Joseph Fletcher, in his book *Morals and Medicine*, declares "an M.D. has a moral obligation to tell the truth, and that withholding it constitutes a deprivation of the patients' rights; therefore it is a theft, therefore unjust, therefore immoral."[61] He further questions whether were the tables turned, the same physicians who practice professional deception would want to be swindled themselves.[62] With this thought in mind, Kant's Categorical Imperative, "Act only on that maxim through which you can at the same time will that it should become a universal law," has definite applicability.[63] A few minutes to consider the Golden Rule and strict practice of it would certainly shed new light on some individual's actions.

The whole concept of placebos and placebo therapy has tremendous relevance to the nursing population. The importance is grounded in the simple fact that while doctors prescribe the placebo, it is often the nurse who commits the observable action of dispensing the preparation. The nurse has the critical task of evaluating her own moral attitudes involved with the practice of deception in placebo therapy. She has a moral obligation to herself and her patient to come to terms with her feelings regarding the practice of such an intervention, and she must be comfortable with that decision. She must have a framework to build her decision upon, and not base her reaction purely on intuition.

Dr. Catherine Murphy, Professor of Nursing at Boston College, has outlined a framework of the nurse-patient relationship that can assist the nurse in recognizing her ethical and moral inclinations. Dr. Murphy describes three separate models, the bureaucratic, the physician advocate, and the patient advocate.[64] The first two models make use of a utilitarian philosophy, where the goal or "good" to be obtained uses the patient and other individuals as means to acquire another end. The bureaucratic model strives to attain an efficiently functioning institution, even if at the patient's or health provider's expense. The physician advocacy model is defined by its paternalistic nature. The physician is omnipotent and a collaborative or collegial relationship with either the patient or the nurse is not encouraged. The third model Dr. Murphy outlines has allegiance to the deontological theory. This model seems most consistent with determination of the nurse's moral choice regarding the use of placebos. The patient advocate model acknowledges that the patient has a right to demand good care and does not have to be subject to the manipulation of health professionals. The patient is viewed as an intelligent, informed consumer who is responsible for his or her own decisions. He or she has dignity, a right to privacy, and a right to be treated with self-respect. The nurse, in this model, is not subservient to the physician or an extension of her or him. She has her own responsibilities and actions. She is not a part of the physician–patient relationship; rather, she has her own relationship with the patient which carries certain responsibilities and obligations. The nurse possesses a moral authority that carries just as much weight as anyone else's, including the physician's. The goal of the patient advocate model is preservation and promotion of individual autonomy, self-actualization, and development of the patient as a unique individual.

If nursing subscribes to the patient advocate model, then the profession must recognize its obligation to protect individuality and foster its growth. The nurse must possess the ethical insight and moral courage to evaluate issues that are presented to her, and as with the case of placebos, this author contends that there is no other conclusion than that placebo therapy constitutes deceptive practice. Nurses have the individual right and moral obligation to decline to involve themselves in such a practice, as it is forbidden by Natural Law and contrary to Kant's Imperative that directs each of us to "act in such a way that you treat humanity, whether in your own person or in the person of any other, never as a means, but always at the same time as an end."[65]

> If it be well weighed, to say that a man lieth is as much to say as that he is brave towards God and a coward towards men. For a lie faces God, and shrinks from man.
>
> Francis Bacon on Truth

> . . . lies beget as a rule, not any acute indignation, but rather a quiet chronic incredulity.
>
> R. C. Cabot on
> Thoughts on the Doctor–Patient Relationship

Endnotes

1. A. K. Shapiro, "Factors Contributing to the Placebo Effect," *American Journal of Psychotherapy* 18 (1964), pp. 73–88.

2. A. K. Shapiro, "The Placebo Effect in the History of Medical Treatment: Implications for Psychiatry," *American Journal of Psychotherapy* 18 (1964), pp. 298–304.
3. *Ibid.*
4. H. M. Adler and V. B. O. Hammett, "The Doctor–Patient Relationship Revisited: An Analysis of the Placebo Effect," *Annals of Internal Medicine* 78 (April 1973), pp. 595–598.
5. S. Bok, *Lying: Moral Choice in Public and Private Life* (New York: Pantheon Books, 1978).
6. *Ibid.*
7. A. O. Berg, "Placebos: A Brief Review for Family Physicians," *Journal of Family Practice* 5, no. 1 (July 1977), pp. 97–100.
8. Shapiro, "The Placebo Effect in the History of Medical Treatment."
9. *Ibid.*
10. *Ibid.*
11. Adler and Hammett, "The Doctor–Patient Relationship."
12. "Letter: Ethics of the Placebo," *British Medical Journal* 1, no. 6007 (February 1976), p. 459.
13. Berg, "Placebos."
14. J. Comaroff, "A Bitter Pill to Swallow: Placebo Therapy in General Practice," *Sociological Review* 24, no. 1 (February 1976), pp. 79–96.
15. C. K. Hofling, "The Place of Placebos in Medical Practice," *General Practitioner* 11, no. 6 (June 1955), pp. 103–107.
16. H. K. Beecher, "The Powerful Placebo," *Journal of the American Medical Association* 159 (December 1955), pp. 1602–1606.
17. O. H. P. Pepper, "A Note on the Placebo," *American Journal of Pharmacology* 117 (1945), pp. 409–412. B. Mead, A. K. Shapiro, and S. Wolf, "Placebo Therapy: When It's a Boon Not a Boondoggle," *Patient Care* 6 (September 1971), pp. 110–111ff. A. Leslie, "Ethics and the Practice of Placebo Therapy," *American Journal of Medicine* 16 (1954), pp. 854–862. Berg, "Placebos."
18. L. Lasagna, "Placebos," *Science American* 193 (1955), pp. 68–71.
19. L. W. Fligor "Letter: The Placebo Effect," *Journal of the American Medical Association* 234, no. 8 (November 1975), p. 808.
20. Lasagna, "Placebos." Mead, Shapiro, and Wolf, "Placebo Therapy."
21. Shapiro, "Factors Contributing to the Placebo Effect." H. Benson and M. D. Epstein, "Patient Consent: What Makes It Informed?" *Drug Information Journal* 9 (March-April 1975), pp. 50–52. M. I. Donovan and S. G. Pierce, *Cancer Care Nursing* (New York: Appleton-Century-Crofts, 1976). Berg, "Placebos." N. Cousins and S. Schiefelbein, "Medical Mystery of the Placebo," *Reader's Digest* 112 (March 1978), pp. 167–169.
22. J. E. Bishop, "Placebos Are Harmless But They Work: Posing Problems for Medicine," *Wall Street Journal*, 25 August 1977.
23. Benson and Epstein, "Patient Consent."
24. D. R. Doongaji, V. N. Vahia, and P. E. Bharucha, "On Placebos, Placebo Responses and Placebo Responders," *Journal of Postgraduate Medicine* 24, no. 2 (April 1978), pp. 91–97.

25. Benson and Epstein, "Patient Consent."
26. H. Brody, *Ethical Dimensions in Medicine* (Boston: Little, Brown, 1976).
27. *Ibid.*
28. A. Fagothey, *Right and Reason* (St. Louis: C. V. Mosby, 1963).
29. G. J. Annas, "The Patient Has Rights. How Can We Protect Them?" *Hastings Center Report* 3 (September 1973), pp. 8–9.
30. S. Vaisrub, "Primum Non Placere?" *Journal of the American Medical Association* 242, no. 3 (July 1979), pp. 276–278.
31. Comaroff, "A Bitter Pill to Swallow," L. Schindel, "The Placebo Dilemma," *European Journal of Clinical Pharmacology* 13, no. 3 (May 1978), pp. 231–235.
32. Comaroff, "A Bitter Pill to Swallow."
33. Shapiro, "The Placebo Effect in the History of Medical Treatment."
34. P. Koeno, "The Placebo Effect in Patent Medicine," *Psychology Today* (April 1974), pp. 60–61.
35. F. Hoff, "The Doctor and His Drug," *Triangle* 6, no. 4 (January 1964), pp. 128–138.
36. S. Bok, "The Ethics of Giving Placebos," *Scientific American* 231 (November 1974), pp. 17–23.
37. T. J. Silber, "Placebo Therapy: The Ethical Dimension," *Journal of the American Medical Association* 242, no. 3 (July 1979), pp. 245–246.
38. A. Meisel, L. H. Roth, and C. W. Liddy, "Toward a Model of the Legal Doctrine of Informed Consent," *American Journal of Psychiatry* 134, no. 3 (March 1977), pp. 285–289.
39. K. Vaux, *Biomedical Ethics* (New York: Harper and Row, 1974).
40. Meisel, Roth, and Liddy, "Toward a Model of the Legal Doctrine of Informed Consent."
41. *Ibid.*, H. W. Foster, "Why Bother With Informed Consent?" *Journal of Medical Education* 52, no. 2 (February 1978), pp. 154–155.
42. R. Schlensky, "Informed Consent and Confidentiality: Proposed New Approaches in Illinois," *American Journal of Psychiatry* 134, no. 12 (December 1977), pp. 1416–1418.
43. G. Sharpe, "Consent to Medical Treatment," *Canadian Medical Association Journal* 117, no. 6 (September 1977), pp. 692–694, 697.
44. *Ibid.*
45. Foster, "Why Bother with Informed Consent?"
46. L. B. Besch, "Informed Consent: A Patient's Right," *Nursing Outlook* 27, no. 1 (January 1979), pp. 32–35.
47. G. J. Annas, "The Hospital: A Human Rights Wasteland," *The Civil Liberties Law Review* (Fall 1974), pp. 9–27.
48. Brody, *Ethical Dimensions in Medicine.*
49. H. Byerly, "Explaining and Exploiting Placebo Effects," *Perspectives in Biology and Medicine* 19 (Spring 1976), pp. 423–436.
50. Bok, "The Ethics of Giving Placebos." Schindel, "The Placebo Dilemma."
51. Bok, *Lying.*
52. J. D. Levine, N. C. Gordon, and H. L. Fields, "The Mechanism of Placebo Analgesia," *Lancet* (September 1978), p. 657.

53. H. K. Beecher, "The Powerful Placebo," *Journal of the American Medical Association* 159 (December 1955), pp. 1602–1606. M. McCaffery, *The Nursing Management of the Patient with Pain* (Philadelphia: Lippincott, 1972).
54. Bok, *Lying.*
55. Bok, "The Ethics of Giving Placebos."
56. Fagothey, *Right and Reason.*
57. *Ibid.*
58. A. J. Davis and M. A. Aroskar, *Ethical Dilemmas and Nursing Practice* (New York: Appleton-Century-Crofts, 1978).
59. F. H. Marsh, "An Ethical Approach to Paternalism in the Physician–Patient Relationship," *Ethics in Science and Medicine* 4, nos. 3–4 (1977), pp. 135–138.
60. Bok, "The Ethics of Giving Placebos."
61. J. Fletcher, *Morals and Medicine* (Boston: Beacon Press, 1954).
62. B. C. Meyer, "Truth and the Physician," *The Bulletin of the New York Academy of Medicine* (January 1969), pp. 59–71.
63. I. Kant, *The Fundamental Principles of the Metaphysic of Morals,* trans. H. J. Patton (New York: Harper Torchbooks, 1948).
64. C. Murphy, "Ethical Aspects of Decision-Making in Nursing," *Political, Social and Educational Forces on Nursing: Impact of Social Forces* (New York: National League for Nursing, 1979).
65. Kant, *The Fundamental Principles of the Metaphysic of Morals.*

Bibliography

Agnew, L. R. "Humanism in Medicine." *Lancet* 2 (1977): 596–598.
Alderman, M. M. "Round Table: Chronic Pain Tactics, which Agent for what Pain Level?" *Patient Care* 12 (1978): 180–181.
Annas, G. J. "Medical Remedies and Human Rights," *Human Rights* 2 (1972): 151–167.
Barnlund, D. C. "The Mystification of Meaning: Doctor–Patient Encounters." *Journal of Medical Education* 51 (1976): 716–725.
Beauchamp, T. L. and Walters, L. *Contemporary Issues in Bioethics.* Encino, Calif.: Dickenson Publishing, 1978.
Beecher, H. *Research and the Individual.* Boston: Little, Brown, 1970.
Bhide, N. K. "Wellington and the Placebo." *British Medical Journal* 2 (1971): 585.
Blackwell, B., Bloomfield, S., and Buncher, C. R. "Demonstration to Medical Students of Placebo Responses and Non-drug Factors. *Lancet* 1 (1972: 1279–1282.
Blackstone, W. T. *Meaning and Existence.* New York: Holt, Rinehart and Winston, 1971.
Brody, H. "The Physician–Patient Contract: Legal and Ethical Aspects." *Journal of Legal Medicine,* July-August 1976, pp. 25–30.

——— . "On Placebos." *Hastings Center Report,* April 1975, pp. 17–18.

Bush, P. J. "The Placebo Effect." *Nursing Digest* 4 (1976): 12–15.

Cabot, R. A. "The Use of Truth and Falsehood in Medicine." *Connecticut Medicine* 42 (1978): 189–194.

Clouser, K. D. "Medical Ethics: Some Uses, Abuses and Limitations." *New England Journal of Medicine* 293 (1975): 384–387.

Collard, J. "A Sociopsychological Approach to the Placebo Effect." *Review Medicine Liege* 32 (1977): 334–339.

Dellinger, A. M. and Warren, D. G. "Frankness in the Doctor–Patient Relationship." *Popular Government,* June 1972, pp. 14–17.

Eck, M. *Lies and Truth.* London: Collier Macmillan, 1970. (Chapter 9)

Englhardt, H. T. "Patient as Person: An Empty Phrase? Four Ethical Problem Areas." *Journal of Texas Medicine* 71 (1975): 57–63.

Fields, H. L. "Secrets of the Placebo." *Psychology Today* 12 (November 1978): 172.

Freedman, B. "A Moral Theory of Informed Consent." *Hastings Center Report* 5 (1975): 32–39.

Herman, J. B. "Placebos." *Prescription Journal* 8 (1969): 84–88.

Henderson, L. J. "Exposition of the Non-utilitarian Argument for Truth-telling. Physician–Patient as a Social System." *New England Journal of Medicine,* 2 May 1935, pp. 819–823.

Jellinek, M. "Erosion of Patient Trust in Large Medical Centers." *Hastings Center Report* 6 (1976): 16–19.

Kabat, E. A. "Ethics and the Wrong Answer." *Science* 189 (1975): 505.

Kadlec, J. F. and Dinno, N. D. "Placebos: A Place in Medical Therapy?" *Journal of the Kentucky Medical Association* 75 (1977): 538–541.

Kao, C. C. L. "Maturity and Paternalism in Health Care." *Ethics in Science and Medicine,* 3 September 1976, pp. 179–186.

Karoly, P. "Ethical Considerations in the Application of Self Control Techniques." *Journal of Abnormal Psychology* 84 (1975): 175–177.

Katz, J. and Cabot, R. C. "Some Reflections on Deception and Placebos in the Practice of Medicine." *Connecticut Medicine* 42 (1978): 199–200.

Kelman, H. C. "Was Deception Justified and Was It Necessary. Comments on Self-control Techniques as an Alternative to Pain Medication." *Journal of Abnormal Psychology* 84 (1975): 172–174.

Korsch, B. M. and Negrete, V. R. "Doctor–Patient Communication." *Scientific American,* August 1972, pp. 66–74.

Lasagna, L. "Further Studies on the Pharmacology of Placebo Administration." *Journal of Clinical Investigation* 37 (1958): 533–537.

Levendusky, P. and Pankratz, L. "Self Control Techniques as an Alternative to Pain Medication." *Journal of Abnormal Psychology* 84 (1975): 165–168.

Lund, C. C. "The Doctor, the Patient, and the Truth." *Annals of Internal Medicine* 24 (1946): 955.

Marriot, I. A. "The Geneva Convention: Humanitarian Law and Medicine." *Canadian Medical Association Journal* 118 (1978): 565–572.

McCaffery, M. *Nursing Management of the Patient with Pain.* Philadelphia: Lippincott, 1972.

Milgran, S. "Subject Reaction: the Neglected Factor in the Ethics of Experimentation." *Hastings Center Report* 1 (1977): 19–23.

Patten, S. C. "Deceiving Subjects (letter)." *Hastings Center Report* 8 (1978): 39.

Pelletier, K. R. *Mind as Slayer, Mind as Healer.* New York: Dell, 1977.

Pogge, R. C. "The Toxic Placebo." *Medical Times* 91 (1963): 773.

Reinhardt, A. and Gray, R. M. "A Social Psychological Study of Attitude Change in Physicians." *Journal of Medical Education* 47 (1972): 112–117.

Ryden, M. G. "An Approach to Ethical Decision-Making." *Nursing Outlook* 26 (1978): 705–706.

Shapiro, A. K. and Strueng, E. L. "The Use of Placebos: A Study of Ethics and Physicians Attitudes." *Psychiatry in Medicine* 4 (1973): 17–29.

Sice, J. "Evaluating Medication." *Lancet* 2 (1972): 651.

Simmons, B. "Problems in Deceptive Medical Procedures: An Ethical and Legal Analysis of the Administration of Placebos." *Journal of Medical Ethics* 4 (1978): 172–181.

Stuntz, R. C. "Informed Consent via Truth Telling and Caring." *Southern Medicine* 63 (1975): 17–22.

Veatch, R. M. "Medical Ethics." *Journal of the American Medical Association* 239 (1978): 514–515.

Vrhovac, B. "Placebo and Its Importance in Medicine." *International Journal of Clinical Pharmacology* 15 (1977): 161–165.

Whalen, D. J. "Clinical Trials: Ethical and Legal Responsibilities of Pharmacists." *Australian Journal of Hospital Pharmacy* 5 (1975): 174.

Wolf, S. "Pharmacology of Placebos." *Pharmacological Review* 11 (1959): 689–703.

Wolff, R. P. *Philosophy: A Modern Encounter.* Englewood Cliffs, N. J.: Prentice-Hall, 1971.

"Truth and Falsehood in Medicine." *Journal of the American Medical Association* 239 (1978): 1554.

"Placebo Effects." *British Medical Journal* 1 (1970): 437.

"Code for Nurses: Ethical Concepts Applied to Nursing." *International Nursing Review* 22 (1975): 8–9.

"Controlled Trials: Planned Deception?" *Lancet* 1 (1979): 534–535.

"Endorphin Update." *Pain* 5 (1978): 3–4.

We have become aware through sensational stories in the public press of the remarkable breakthroughs in the development of life-prolonging—or is it death-delaying—machines. We have also become aware of the problems such machines present: who shall receive their benefits, who shall determine when the time has come to turn them off and let the patient die without further intervention, who shall pay the enormous costs when a given patient is not able to do so? We have not, however, been made aware of the moral and ethical problems facing the professional nurse within this context. The following essay by Linda O'Brien offers a thoughtful examination of the problems raised for nurses in the allocation of a scarce resource. She focuses on a particular case involving the transplantation of bone marrow. Her extensive consideration of the alternatives facing decision makers in such cases and her review of the opinions of a number of commentators in this field demonstrate effectively that the nursing professional has a contribution to make and an obligation to be heard in this complex and increasingly often encountered problem.

15

Allocation of a Scarce Resource: The Bone Marrow Transplant Case

Linda O'Brien

Technology has increased today to such a great degree that it is possible to extend the life of a dying person by treating her or him with a life-saving measure so complex that we may call it exotic. Along with great feats of biomedical ingenuity comes the problem of allocating such exotic life-saving measures. The allocation of the life-saving treatment becomes a problem or dilemma because the treatment costs a great deal of money, time, and labor which could, and perhaps should, be spent elsewhere.

Health care costs are rising all the time along with spiraling inflation. To control these costs the federal government has instituted some measures to help the consumer of health care in certain cases, such as the catastrophic end-stage renal disease. Now other terminal conditions require last-chance treatment also, but the governmental agencies have not been so generous in distributing the needed resources. Perhaps the agencies have recognized the tremendous financial burden the end-stage renal program has placed on them. The end-stage renal program expanded. As the need for it increased, there was an increase in the number of renal dialysis units. Other exotic life-saving measures have not been so widely distributed even though the demand for them has increased. When the demand exceeds the supply, we have what is termed a scarce resource. Scarce resources are allocated to certain hospitals or institutions which indicate that they can provide them to the greatest number of people in the greatest need. When only a few institutions are given the resources or when the demand exceeds the supply, one is describing *macroallocation*, the first step in distributing a scarce resource.[1]

Macroallocation means that only a small number of institutions (or persons in the case of research funding) get the funds to provide the treatment or do the research in a specific area. Macroallocation of an exotic life-saving treatment becomes a problem because, although the need for the resource increases, the need for other health care resources in the health care delivery system is greater. The cries for other types of health care needs, especially basic needs by a larger number of persons, help to control and keep down the allocation of an exotic life-saving measure demanded by few.

Once the scarce resource has been distributed to a specific institution, a second problem, which is much more commonly seen by nurses, arises. This is the problem of who shall receive the scarce resource. When one is discussing distribution of the resource for needy patients, one is then focusing on *micro-allocation.*[2] Problems of microallocation come up frequently in our nursing practice. We have to make decisions about who gets the last bed in the intensive care unit if several patients are in very critical condition and could use it. Who gets to use the last Stryker frame bed when several patients could benefit from it? Who gets the corneal transplant when more than one patient matches for it? These are but a few of the problems we face.

These types of situations are considered problems of microallocation because they focus on the distribution of the resource such as a treatment, a piece of equipment, a drug or procedure to a specific individual in need. These problems arise constantly and the decisions made to solve them are usually not made randomly; instead, some quick assessment of risks versus benefits is made, usually with little emphasis placed on ethical principles of equality. When not all can have an opportunity to have the scarce resource, who shall have the resource and who decides becomes a real dilemma. Decision making approaches for scarce resources involve many ethical principles and reveal that there are various viewpoints on the subject. Some of the most common views on the distribution of a scarce resource are these: to extend treatment to no one, to treat someone by random selection, and to treat someone with reference to whether the patient meets some established criteria.[3]

There are several major considerations relating to the problem of an exotic life-saving treatment: macroallocation, microallocation, cost, biomedical ingenuity, and decision making. All of these concepts also relate to the major theme of a case to be presented in this paper, that of *distributive justice.* Distributive justice means exactly what the words imply, distributing the goods (a scarce resource) justly and fairly.[4] Justice is relative to the time and place or framework in which a person works. In the United States one is sent to jail and pays a fine if caught stealing, but in the Middle East one may have one's hand cut off. The price for the crime is different depending on the orientation or system one is living in. Many would defend both types of systems of social justice depending on each person's orientation. Justice in health care is not exactly an issue of social justice (although some identify it as such), but is definitely an issue in distributive justice, and, depending on one's orientation, the operation of the system differs. An example of differences in orientation is the end-stage renal program. In the United States all victims of this disease have treatment provided for them; in the United Kingdom all do not.[5] Arguments for both types of systems can be supported depending on one's orientation.

One's orientation must be considered because health care distribution in this country is a result of a concern to cure rather than to prevent disease. In the case of terminal illness, the search for a cure has led us to provide exotic life-saving measures that can prolong one's life. This "curing orientation" can exhaust funds in caring for a very small population of dying people. To prevent exhausting the funds and still be just in distributing the treatment, one looks for alternative methods for distributing the scarce resource. The case in this paper presents the problem of distributing the scarce resource. It raises several principles of justice and related issues of ethical philosophy. Both positive and negative viewpoints concerning different approaches to distributing a scarce resource will be discussed. The scarce resource in this case is the use of a life-island for bone marrow transplant and the special team that goes along with the life-island.

N. E. was a twenty-one-year-old unmarried mother when she was admitted to the intensive care unit for isolation. She had noticed frequent bruising on her legs and a persistent sore throat. Due to her recent reading from medical texts, she came to the hospital questioning the possibility of leukemia. She was correct, a diagnosis of AML (Acute Myelocytic Leukemia) was made.

She was five months pregnant on admission and it was feared that the chemotherapy drugs that she needed crossed the placenta, damaging the unborn child. After much discussion, the pregnancy was terminated. R., the father of their one-year-old daughter, and her mother were continual sources of support.

The treatment was painful; and N. E. cried and screamed with each blood transfusion and the chemotherapy administration. She developed phlebitis, her skin sloughed, she developed mouth ulcers and nasal bleeding. Strict isolation technique was required, as her white blood cell count would drop below 700.

After many weeks, N. E. was discharged in remission. She was readmitted several times during the year for spontaneous nasal bleeding or vaginal bleeding, but returned home each time to be with R. and care for A., their daughter. R. worked infrequently, and N. E. received welfare to support the family.

One year after her initial hospital contact, N. E. had an exacerbation of her AML. The hematology staff suggested a bone marrow transplant. Although the hospital staff could have performed such an operation, it was felt that success of the procedure would be improved by sending N. E. either to Seattle, where there was a transplant service for leukemics, or to another hospital in Boston, which had a "life-island," an isolation unit that eliminated bacteria by laminar flow. The life-island had been funded through a National Institute of Health grant as a clinical study unit. N. E.'s sister was typed as a suitable donor, however, the cross-match had missed Seattle's criteria for acceptance by one factor.

She was accepted in Boston at the same time another patient was diagnosed with AML within the hospital in which the island was located. The Research Committee decided to delay N. E. as they chose to transplant one of their own patients first, before accepting a transfer. She would have had to wait one month.

During that month, N. E.'s white blood cells and platelet count dropped dramatically. She began to bleed from various bodily orifices. Her mouth was ulcerated and her breath uncomfortable from bleeding and crusts. She was bruised everywhere, especially in the face, which swelled, forcing her eyes closed. In this state, she remained alert, serving as a source of strength to those close to her.

N. E. died early one afternoon, two weeks before her scheduled surgery.

The clinical picture is typical of a patient with leukemia. N. E. had all of the possible treatments available to her in the hospital setting except one, the bone marrow transplant. The bone marrow transplant was her last alternative available for life. The number of transplants done today with complete success of long-term survival is still minimal and the number of hospitals that even offer transplant as an alternative is very small.[6] Of those hospitals that do provide the transplant treatment only a few have a "life-island" apparatus which gives the patient a greater chance of survival.

The opportunity for the bone marrow transplant is considered a scarce resource for two reasons: very few institutions offer this procedure and the possibility for donors is limited to immediate family members. N. E. was fortunate enough to have at least one institution available to her for the procedure and had a viable donor.

The data available to this writer do not present other persons who have requested this scarce resource at the same time. In such circumstances where one person has been denied treatment, it would be desireable for the public to have full knowledge of this situation because it would test the principle of equality of health care and could affect public policy. Some authors feel that this type of situation legally resembles the "life-boat" incidents of the Titanic, but on a small scale.[7] In the case of the Titanic many innocent lives were not saved and the question of whose life should have been saved still exists today.

Some psychosocial considerations in this case worth noting are: if N. E. dies by not having transplant treatment, she will leave a child parentless; N. E. is only twenty-one years old and the other candidate is forty years old; N. E. could suffer psychological stress if social worth criteria judged her non-valuable. In order to consider age a factor in the decision-making process, one should know more about the other candidate, but if nothing else is known one may see that N. E. is considerably younger and perhaps like a child compared to a forty-year-old-candidate. Many people would prefer to try to save the younger generation and in this case may have preferred N. E. to the forty-year-old person.

Much research in the area of maternal-child bonding would also call attention to the danger of not trying to preserve the mother of a young child. This research clearly indicates that separation of the child from the mother can cause emotional scarring in the child which may last throughout its life.[8] In order to prevent this problem one could emphasize that by trying to save N. E. one was also trying to save an innocent child from becoming emotionally scarred.

Another psychosocial consideration of stress as a result of being rejected by the committee because of social worth did not occur in this case. N. E. and the forty-year-old candidate were not compared on the social worth criteria, thus N. E. did not have this pressure added on to her already debilitated condition.

According to a nurse who was on the committee considering both candidates, N. E. was a better candidate by one factor for the Boston transplant unit. Even though N. E. was a more medically acceptable candidate, the later patient was taken because she already had made previous connections with this institution. Her access was given priority on the principle of first come, first serve.

Nursing care of N. E. would not differ dramatically from care of the forty-year-old candidate. One of the nurses who has managed the care of previous patients in the life-island has indicated that adult patients are generally more difficult to care for than children. Adults get bored and become psychotic more quickly and easily than children. Since both of the patients being considered were adults, the nursing care would essentially be the same, that of care for an adult patient within a confined environment.

One of the problems with nursing care of a patient in this environment is that of long-term isolation without human contact. Sometimes the transplant takes a long time for acceptance or a long time before complete rejection is confirmed. One might propose administration of a psychological examination as to which candidate could best tolerate this type of isolation. This could be one criterion for determining who should be treated. In this case no one considered this type of criterion, and perhaps most people would consider this totally inappropriate, but I feel that it should be put on the table for a complete examination of the psychosocial aspects of this case in conjunction with the nursing considerations.

Another problem with the care of patients who receive a bone marrow transplant is the devastating side effects. Such patients undergo a complete radiation of their entire body which causes severe prolonged diarrhea, mouth ulcers with bleeding, anorexia, and severe pain. In fact, these side effects are so devastating that the institution has stopped the transplant program because it was considered cruel as well as ineffectual.

The last consideration about this case is the cost. The life-island was considered very expensive when the program first started many years ago, and costs have steadily increased. A bone marrow transplant costs the consumer huge sums of money which are not paid by the patient but by federal money. The total operation of the transplant team and unit maintenance cannot be estimated by looking at dollars and cents alone. The total cost has to be viewed in terms of money, time, and valuable energy.

Several ethical issues, such as distributive justice, quality of life, human experimentation, informed consent, and, lastly, privacy of the patient, are involved in this case. Each one of these issues will be addressed to some extent, but the issue of distributive justice will be discussed in more detail.

N. E. is a terminally ill person and has almost no chance for survival even with this treatment. Some would not advocate prolonging the life of such a person if the method would entail debilitating side effects. More suffering for the sake of saving a person by means of an exotic life-saving measure does not preserve the quality of the life already present. In order to preserve the social and personal dignity of a person one should not offer such harmfully devastating treatments but work to make death a peaceful event.

Others advocate that as long as a person has neocortical functioning, he or she is human and deserves all possible chances for life or survival.[9] N. E. never lost neocortical functioning and therefore should have been given every opportunity for life and survival.

Human experimentation is an ethical issue in this case because the patient is considered a study subject. She is a study subject because the life-island is supported by a federal grant. The patient has no choice about whether she wants to be part of a human experimentation project because this treatment is considered experimental in nature.

Hans Jonas notes that one has two ways of looking at the problem of human experimentation. The first way is that of therapeutic experimentation and the other is non-therapeutic experimentation. In therapeutic experimentation the doctor only proposes the treatment to a patient if the patient could benefit from it. In the therapeutic type the experimentation is usually the last alternative for survival and if the patient has exhausted all other conventional treatments the doctor is justified in proposing experimental treatment.[10]

According to Jonas, the type of treatment that the doctor proposes to the patient because nothing conventional is left cannot be justified on the basis that it would assist the doctors in better treating other patients.[11] Experimentation for purpose of clarification of scientific methods and techniques which will be used in the future (future orientation) cannot be approved because the patient is treated as a means to an end. To be treated as a means to an end for the purpose of improving the conditions of others and not the patient reduces the patient's worth as a human and defies the Kantian principle "never treat people as a means to an end."[12] In this case, N. E.'s doctor only proposed the transplant because he thought it would help her.

One must consider the issue of informed consent in this case because the procedure presents many risks to a patient. The greater the risk the more information a patient needs in order to give consent freely. In the free enterprise system the consumer is given information about a material good before the purchase. If the information has been misleading or not correct, one has means for exchange, and laws protect the person from fraud. In the case of a bone marrow transplant, no exchange system can apply; therefore, one needs total and unbiased information before a decision can be made. Beauchamp and Walters point out that "the ability to make a decision is largely dependent upon the information made available to the patient and that a patient's consent to a medical procedure would be insignificant if important relevant information were withheld."[13]

In this case N. E. was not given full information about exactly what the treatment entailed, especially about the devastating side effects. This information was purposely withheld because the team felt that this information would deter her or any other patient from receiving treatment. Also, this patient was not given full information about the rate of survival, nor that survival is considered merely one hundred days of life after termination of treatment. It can be seen that withholding information has some benefits for those providing the treatment and has some benefits to the patient in that the treatment may help the patient. But by not totally informing the patient one is not truly getting informed consent, and in the case of N. E., her agreement to accept treatment is not valid because she was not totally informed.

The Patient's Bill of Rights states that "A patient has the right to every consideration of his privacy concerning his own medical care program. Case discussion, consultation, examination, and treatment are confidential and should be conducted discreetly. Those not directly involved in his care must have permission of the patient to be present."[14] Information from a member of the transplant team indicates to us that in this case the patient's right to privacy cannot be assured by this institution. Her privacy would be violated because she is a research subject and open to investigation. Since the life-island is a medical novelty and a learning experience for those in the health care field, the patient is exposed to numerous inquiries as well as observation. Since this patient has no chance for total privacy, one can agree that N. E. is a victim of scientific advancement and reduced to an object status like a means to an end. In this case N. E. jeopardizes her patient status and loses her privacy right by accepting this treatment.

N. E.'s case is a problem of microallocation. The life-island at this hospital can only be used by one patient at a time. Two questions arise out of this situation: should N. E. have equal access to health care (use of the life-island), and how does one decide whether equal access measures are being used? Answers to these questions are usually based on one of three main principles of distributive justice:[15]

1. Justice is dealing with people according to their deserts or merits.
2. Justice is treating human beings as equals in the sense of distributing good and evil equally among them.
3. Justice is treating people according to their needs or abilities or both.

The first principle is considered the classical meritorious criterion of justice, the second is characteristic of modern democratic society, and the third is associated more with Marxist philosophy.

Frankena points out that distribution according to merit or virtue would be immoral because not everyone has an equal chance of achieving virtue or merit. Virtue can only be considered the basis of distribution if the conditions in society are equally distributed, thus allowing merit or virtue to be distinguished.[16] Frankena also indicates that to distribute according to needs and abilities would also be unjust and immoral because everyone does not have the same abilities and needs. A system that would proportion the goods according to abilities would surely punish those who do not have abilities, such as some handicapped persons, but who have needs as great as or greater than many others.[17] Frankena points out that the second principle based on egalitarian philosophy is a *prima facie* rule, calling for equal treatment for all.

Even though Frankena argues that equal treatment for all should be the ruling principle, he does feel that on occasion the *prima facie* rule can be superseded by a higher principle which is beneficence. He states,

> We may claim, however, that in distributing the goods, evil, help, tasks, roles, and so forth, people are to be treated equally in the sense indicated, except when unequal treatment can be justified by the consideration of beneficence (including utility) or on the ground that it will promote greater equality in the long run. Unequal treatment always requires justification and only certain kinds of justification suffice.[18]

Frankena supports equal treatment in most cases unless some other relevant factors come into play. His support for utility in the arguments for distribution gives some justification to utility as a criterion for allocating a scarce resource. Since the principle of beneficence can also be considered in distributive justice of a scarce resource, the problem of allocation is complex and difficult to handle.

Distribution of a scarce resource can be achieved in several ways according to the principles of distributive justice. First, giving no one treatment ensures equal treatment for all. Second, treatment may be based on an established selection system. The selection system can be either a complex criteria system, where both medical acceptability and social worth are considered, or a random system where everyone has an equal chance.[19] A third alternative is to have a system that treats all persons in need. In this system one would also be ensuring equal treatment for all.

The second alternative, especially the complex criteria formula, seems to use distributive justice with the principle of beneficence added to it. With the complex criteria system, the person in need is evaluated according to medical acceptability (relative likelihood of success, and life-expectancy factors) and according to social worth (family role factor, potential future contribution factor, and past contribution factor).[20] Let us consider these alternatives and weigh the positive and negative aspects of each of them.

Edmond Cahn addresses the question "who shall live when not all can live?" His answer is "no one." He points out that to give treatment to some persons and not to all is morally wrong because those who do not get the treatment have been programmed for death. It is morally wrong to take the life of an innocent person, and giving treatment to one person and not another causes the death of an innocent person.[21]

Advocates of a minimum health care program find it morally unacceptable to use funds to provide exotic life-saving treatment to a few people.[22] Charles Fried, for example, feels that health care is a right, but that right does not entail a maximum distribution of health care to everyone. Another supporter for minimum health care and not treatment for each and every disease is Leon Kass. Kass points out that the end-stage renal program has violated the national interest because funds which could provide basic care to many are used to provide long-term care for few.[23] Since both of these scholars advocate minimum health care as a right, I assume both would see it as immoral to provide exotic life-saving treatment to few. In their view, exotic life-saving treatment to few violates the principle of equality and of minimum health care for all.

Since most theorists advocate that some type of system be established to select who gets treatment when not all can have treatment, it appears they support the idea of treatment for someone and do not support treatment for no one. Their support for treatment for at least some persons is expressed by Childress when he says "letting everyone die is not good either."[24] This statement reflects the idea that to let everyone die would be an irresponsible way to handle a scarce resource.

If no one got the treatment, we would never be able to experiment and find a cure. We need to remember that to enhance and promote curing one has to take the risk-benefit steps that both science and technology call for. If we had not taken those steps in trying to treat polio, we would still have iron-lung wards today. A certain amount of human experimentation is necessary and beneficial for humanity.

The last argument for treatment is that in the Hippocratic oath the doctor makes a statement that she or he will try to treat all her or his patients in the best way possible. If a treatment is possible, does a doctor have the right to refuse this treatment to a patient if it can help him or her? One would assume that, as long as some treatment is available, the doctor has an obligation to offer it to some patient who could benefit from it.

The selection process is one of the most complicated yet popular alternatives. It is complicated because strong arguments for both methods proposed in this system have strong support. Some support random selection. This may be a "first come, first serve" or a lottery system. Others support a complex criteria system which has been described previously. Let us consider arguments for and against both the lottery and the complex criteria system involving medical acceptability and social worth criteria.

There are a number of reasons for supporting a lottery system of access to health care. It preserves the principle of equality of access by denying any criterion for such access other than random chance. If one argues that each person has a right to equality, it is necessary that equal access be available for any given resource. As the need for health care is universal, equality of distribution of the resource of health care is required.

The random selection or lottery system preserves each person's dignity and worth. It avoids the dilemma of having a situation in which one person must be the judge of another person's worthiness to receive social and medical resources. A lottery system assures that no one has an unfair advantage for access to health care.

Some advocates of the lottery hold that it follows the natural law of God. Good and evil come to all people and no one can know how God makes decisions. The lottery assures that no person will play God and make decisions concerning life and death matters.[25]

Use of the lottery prevents one from using a "productiveness" type of criterion for judgment purposes. The criterion of productiveness in the past or likelihood in the future would eliminate both very young and very old people because persons in each group would not meet either requirement. A young child has no past contributions to reflect upon and an elderly person may not be able to guarantee future contributions.

The lottery follows one of the principles of social justice that is "equal treatment for similar cases."[26] This principle of justice is identified as a strong supportive principle of equal access to the resource in similar cases as, for example, all who have terminal leukemia, all need the transplant.

The lottery preserves the doctor–patient relationship.[27] If the patient were told by her or his doctor that she or he was not worthy of treatment, the patient might lose all hope and will to live. The patient might lose trust in the entire health care profession. It would be morally wrong to allow a patient to lose dignity as a person or to shatter a trusting relationship by using social worth or medical acceptability as a determining factor in health care delivery.

On the other hand, many theorists oppose the random selection theory. The lottery system does not consider one important point of justice which is "entitlement." Justice requires that the differing circumstances of individual's lives be taken into account when the matter of entitlement to health care is under consideration. In the lottery or random selection theory such circumstances cannot be taken into account and thus an injustice may result.

Another strong argument against the lottery system is that it is an irresponsible way of handling a scarce resource. John Harris points out that "living and dying should not be left to chance because in other areas of human life we believe that we have an obligation to insure survival of the maximum number of lives possible."[28] He is saying that we always try to incorporate systems that protect the greatest number of people; therefore, in the health care system, how can a system which does not assure survival to the greatest number be consistent with present-day thinking? It is irresponsible to put into a lottery those patients who do not have a chance of surviving the treatment (medical acceptability) and thus cut off and reduce the chances of those who would survive the treatment. It appears that John Harris mainly objects to social worth criteria and not medical worth criteria.

Turning to the second selection process, we shall consider first the positive and then the negative positions. Some suggest that the principle of orthodox utilitarianism can be used to support the use of complex criteria. This principle suggests that "a civilized society has the obligation to promote furtherance of an achievement of the culture and other related areas even if certain burdens are assumed."[29] This statement reflects the idea that if the continuation of humankind is to be assured, one needs to take into account certain social worth variables. Thus, a complex criteria system is appropriate.

Nicholas Rescher also supports the complex criteria system because it would be a more responsible way of handling a scarce resource.[30] In the lottery system only one factor, need, was being considered, but in the complex criteria many other factors would be considered and these factors would not reflect the patient's need as much as the need of others. Here beneficence is involved.

Leo Shatin also supports a complex criteria system because he feels that in most medical decision making processes one is always using, consciously or not, some material worth criteria, thus it is engrained into our thinking process.[31]

In general, the strongest supporters of complex criteria argue that a scarce resource should be distributed to those who have the best chance to use it and to survive the treatment. They hold that the treatment should be given to those who need to exist for the benefit of others as well as for humanity. The idea of giving the resource to those who could best survive would be following the Darwinian principle of "survival of the fittest." The latter concept would be supported by the utilitarian principle of beneficence.

Against the use of complex criteria a number of scholars have presented a variety of arguments. A social worth criteria would be very hard to institute because each person has his or her own value system. A universal value system would be nearly impossible to create and, if created, to defend.

Childress observes that to use some social worth criteria can reduce a person's dignity.[32] Many advocates of the lottery system point out that the idea of the patient's "utility" is psychologically damaging to the person. A person is a biological, psychological, and social being with individual worth which should not be judged by anyone other than God.

A final alternative distribution system is to provide transplants to all of those patients who desire them. One does not find support for this position in the literature, but nevertheless some basic supporting arguments for it may be suggested.

If all people who required or desired bone marrow transplants were given the opportunity to have one, one could say that the principle of equality was being practiced. The principles of equal treatment for similar cases as well as equal access to a resource would be followed. If all people who desired treatment received it then the transplant procedure and life-island would not even be an issue of a scarce resource. If services were provided for everyone who desired them, no one would use deviant means, such as offering bribes to members of a complex criteria committee, to acquire them.

Against the idea of giving bone marrow transplants to everyone needing them are a number of considerations. If all patients who wanted a transplant were given one, funds for other special treatment procedures would be depleted. It would be immoral to distribute the goods totally to one group, because other groups would suffer from inequality. In terms of equal distribution one cannot look at the needs of a single group, but must look at the needs of all groups requesting support.

If exotic life-saving measures were distributed in order to prolong the life of dying persons, one would not be contributing to prevention of disease. One must weigh the social and personal implications of helping a population of dying which is limited, while a large population of living exists. There is an obligation to the living that is stronger than to the dying, and therefore less time, energy, and labor should be utilized in prolongation measures for the dying. Lastly, if all patients who desired treatment got it, one would be observing endless human experimentation first-hand.

In conclusion, the complex criteria method which has been suggested by Nicholas Rescher may be seen as especially valuable.[33] He suggests a three-way system which involves medical acceptability, social worth, and lottery. This system would insure that those eligible for the procedure would have an equal chance for treatment. Those who were not eligible would not be considered because they lacked medical acceptability or social worth.

In the present writer's view, it is imperative that treatment be provided to those who would benefit the most, such as those who have the greatest chance to survive. The social worth criteria could be modified in one way. A child up to the age of twenty-one would automatically be acceptable in terms of social worth. Anyone over the age of twenty-one would be reviewed in terms of social worth criteria. Any child that meets the medical acceptability criteria should automatically pass the social worth criteria because a young child or teenager cannot be judged by past contributions. Also a young child can contribute to society in some way in the future and that potential should be recognized. A twenty-two-year-old person is still quite young to have accumulated past contributions, but there has to be a cut-off somewhere.

Rescher's plan should be modified for the young because in our American culture the child is valued highly. Therefore, this idea is consistent with our culture. Also, most young children do better with transplants than adults, and for that reason excluding them as potential candidates on the basis of social worth is unjustified.

If this system were adopted, more transplant units would be needed. More units does not mean that one should reduce money spent for other diseases or research. To have more units means that there should be a regional system similar to that by which neonatal units are made available. Two or three or more states should get together to have one transplant unit available for their constituents. These groups of states could assess their needs and then have a plan that proportions the funding among the users. To have a transplant unit in only Seattle and Boston and perhaps a few other places is not feasible for many patients.

This system would cost the consumer more money, but the consumer is vitally interested in curing diseases. The only way to promote curing is to have more experimentation on those who would be able to survive the treatment. Twenty years from now transplants may be more successful. To insure we reach that success, more transplant centers for patients who could benefit should be available.

This approach indicates that more money should be spent on treatment for persons who need exotic life-saving measures. Such life-saving measures should be more available, but only to those who could best use them, and their use should not be left up to chance. The issues of equality should not be the primary consideration with health care when exotic life-saving measures are being considered. Equal access to a basic minimum of care should be a right, but that right does not apply to exotic life-saving measures. Such life-saving measures call for use of the principle of beneficence which may be regarded as a higher principle than equality.

Endnotes

1. Tom L. Beauchamp and LeRoy Walters, "Part IV: Allocation of Scarce Medical Resources," *Contemporary Issues in Bioethics,* ed. T. L. Beauchamp and LeRoy Walters (Encino, Calif.: Dickenson Publishing, 1978), p. 347.
2. *Ibid.,* p. 349.
3. *Ibid.,* p. 350.
4. William K. Frankena, *Ethics,* 2nd Edition, (Englewood Cliffs, N. J.: Prentice-Hall, 1973), p. 49.
5. Wicard J. H. Mooney, "What is the Monetary Value of Life?" *British Medical Journal,* 1977, p. 1628.
6. Advisory Committee of the Bone Marrow Transplant Registry, "Bone Marrow Transplantation from Donors with Aplastic Anemia." *Journal of the American Medical Association* 236, no. 10 (6 September 1976), p. 1131.
7. Daniel Callahan, "Doing Well by Doing Good: Garrett Hardin's 'Life Boat Ethics,'" *Hastings Center Report,* (December 1974), p. 1.
8. Linda O'Brien, unpublished paper on Maternal-Infant Attachment, Fall, 1978, for Early Parenting Course at Boston University, Boston, Massachusetts.
9. Joseph F. Fletcher, "Four Indicators of Humanhood—The Enquiry Matures." *Hastings Center Report* (December 1974), p. 5.
10. Hans Jonas, "Philosophical Reflections on Experimenting with Human Subjects," *Contemporary Issues in Bioethics,* ed. Tom L. Beauchamp and LeRoy Walters (Encino, Calif.: Dickenson Publishing, 1978), p. 419.

11. *Ibid.,* p. 419.
12. Immanuel Kant, "Categorical Imperative" in P. W. Taylor, *Principles of Ethics* (Encino, Calif.: Dickenson, 1975).
13. Tom L. Beauchamp and LeRoy Walters, *Contemporary Issues in Bioethics,* p. 133.
14. Patient's Bill of Rights. (Chicago: American Hospital Association, 1972).
15. Frankena, *Ethics,* p. 49.
16. *Ibid.,* p. 50.
17. *Ibid.,* p. 51.
18. *Ibid.,* p. 52.
19. Tom L. Beauchamp and LeRoy Walters, "Allocation of Scarce Medical Resources," *Contemporary Issues in Bioethics,* p. 350.
20. *Ibid.,* p. 350.
21. Edmond Cahn, *The Moral Decision* (Bloomington, Ind.: University of Indiana Press, 1974), p. 71.
22. Charles Fried, "Equality and Rights in Medical Care," *Contemporary Issues in Bioethics,* p. 364.
23. Leon R. Kass, "The Pursuit of Health and the Right to Health," *Contemporary Issues in Bioethics,* p. 371.
24. James F. Childress, "Who Shall Live When Not All Can Live?" *Contemporary Issues in Bioethics,* p. 391.
25. John Harris, "The Survival Lottery," *Philosophy* 50 (1975), p. 84.
26. Gene Outka, "Social Justice and Equal Access to Health Care," *Contemporary Issues in Bioethics,* p. 352.
27. Harris, "The Survival Lottery," p. 82.
28. *Ibid.*
29. Nicholas Rescher, "The Allocation of Exotic Medical Lifesaving Therapy," *Contemporary Issues in Bioethics,* p. 383.
30. *Ibid.,* p. 380.
31. Leo Shatin, "Medical Care and the Social Worth of a Man," *American Journal of Orthopsychiatry* 36 (1967), pp. 96–101.
32. Childress, "Who Shall Live. . . ?"
33. Rescher, "Allocation of Exotic Medical Lifesaving Technology," p. 387.

Selected Bibliography

Advisory Committee of the Bone Marrow Transplant Registry. "Bone Marrow Transplantation from Donors with Aplastic Anemia." *Journal of the American Medical Association,* pp. 1131–1135.
Beauchamp, Thomas L. and Walters, LeRoy. *Contemporary Issues in Bioethics.* Encino, Calif.: Dickenson Publishing, 1978.
Blackstone, William T. "On Health Care as a Legal Right—An Exploration of Legal and Moral Grounds. *Georgia Law Review* 10 (1976): 391–418.

Callahan, Daniel. "Doing Well by Doing Good, Garrett Hardin's 'Life Boat Ethics.'" *Hastings Center Report,* December 1976, pp. 1–4.

Callahan, Daniel. "Science: Limits and Prohibitions." *Hastings Center Report,* November 1973, pp. 5–7.

Childress, James F. "Who Shall Live When Not All Can Live?" *Contemporary Issues in Bioethics,* ed. Tom L. Beauchamp and LeRoy Walters. Encino, Calif.: Dickenson Publishing, 1978, pp. 389–398.

Fletcher, Joseph F. "Four Indicators of Humanhood—The Enquiry Matures." *Hastings Center Report,* December 1974, pp. 4–7.

Frankena, William K. *Ethics,* 2nd Edition. Englewood Cliffs, N. J.: Prentice-Hall, 1973, pp. 34–59.

Frankena, William, K. "The Nature of Social Justice" in *Moral Problems in Medicine,* ed. Samuel Gorovitz, *et al.* Englewood Cliffs, N. J.: Prentice-Hall, 1976, pp. 430–443.

Fried, Charles. "Equality and Rights in Medical Care." *Hastings Center Report,* February 1976, pp. 29–36.

Fuchs, Victor R. *Who Shall Live? Health, Economics and Social Choice,* New York: Basic Books, 1974. (Chapters 1, 2, 3, 4, 6).

Harris, John. "The Survival Lottery." *Philosophy* 50 (1978): 81–87.

Hippocratic Oath. *Contemporary Issues in Bioethics,* p. 138.

Jonas, Hans. "Philosophical Reflections on Experimenting with Human Subjects." *Contemporary Issues in Bioethics,* pp. 411–420.

Kass, Leon. "The Pursuit of Health and the Right to Health." *Contemporary Issues in Bioethics,* pp. 371–388.

Levine, Melvin D. M. D., Camital, Bruce, Nathan, David, and Curran, William, "The Medical Ethics of Bone Marrow Transplantation in Childhood." *Journal of Pediatrics* 86 (January 1975): 145–150.

Macklin, Ruth. "Moral Concerns and Appeals to Rights and Duties." *Hastings Center Report,* October 1976, pp. 31–38.

Morillo, Carolyn R. "As Sure as Shooting." *Philosophy* 51:80–89.

Morison, Robert S. "Rights, Responsibility: Redressing the Uneasy Balance." *Hastings Center Report,* April 1974, pp. 1–4.

Mooney, Wicard G. H. "What is the Monetary Value of Life?" *British Medical Journal* 2 (1977): 1627–29.

Ogletree, Thomas W. "Values, Obligations and Virtues—Approaches to Biomedical Ethics." *Journal of Religious Ethics* 4 (1976): 105–30.

Outka, Gene. "Social Justice and Equal Access to Health Care." *Contemporary Issues in Bioethics,* pp. 352–363.

"Patient's Bill of Rights." Chicago: American Hospital Association, 1972.

Rescher, Nicholas. "The Allocation of Exotic Lifesaving Therapy." *Contemporary Issues in Bioethics,* pp. 378–388.

Schiffer, R. B. "Commentary on Case Study in Bioethics: The Last Bed in the ICU." *Hastings Center Report,* December 1977, pp. 21–22.

Shapiro, Michael. "Who Merits Merit? Problems in Distributive Justice and Utility Posed by New Biology." *Southern California Law Review* 48 (1974): 318–370.

Sparer, Edward V. "The Legal Right to Health Care: Public Policy and Equal Access." *Hastings Center Report,* October 1976, pp. 39–46.

Taylor, Vincent. "How Much is Good Health Worth?" *Policy Science* 1 (1970): 49–72.

Telfer, Elizabeth. "Justice, Welfare and Health Care." *Journal of Medical Ethics,* September 1976, pp. 107–111.

The progress of the medical profession toward the goal of more effective treatment of disease sometimes requires the use of human beings as subjects of medical experiments. Such experimentation with human subjects presents basic moral and ethical problems not only to the medical researcher and to the person upon whom the experiment is being carried out but to the nurse and the nursing profession as well. What should the nurse do when she is involved in the administering of experimental medication? By what guidelines does the nurse make her decision regarding her proper role when experiments are being carried out with or without informed consent of the patients involved?

Sandra Reed Sweezy presents in the following essay a nursing perspective on an occasion of medical experimentation with human subjects which gained considerable attention because of its seriousness and complexity. She relates the events at Willowbrook State Hospital in which the subjects of medical experimentation were children. She discusses what was done at Willowbrook, examines implications of decisions made there, and concludes that while research to improve medical care is a desirable enterprise, great care must be taken never to use a patient as a means to an end.

16

The Ethical Issue of Informed Consent in Human Experimentation

Sandra Reed Sweezy

From 1956 to 1970 at Willowbrook State Hospital on Staten Island, New York, more than seven thousand children were placed in a research unit as subjects of studies concerning hepatitis and possible immunization against it.[1] A consultant in pediatrics and infectious disease at the state school, Dr. Saul Krugman, noticed that certain diseases were prevalent at Willowbrook and began a number of studies of them. In one of these studies he researched infectious and serum hepatitis in order to learn about the diseases in general, and also to try to develop methods of immunization. To achieve this goal, it was decided to expose some children to the Willowbrook strain of hepatitis virus in an attempt to achieve controlled conditions for testing a vaccine, namely gamma globulin.[2] The procedures utilized and the findings regarding them have been widely studied. The problems they raise are the subject of this paper, especially as they relate to the ethical issues posed to the nursing profession.

Certain aspects of the Willowbrook hepatitis studies must be presented before a detailed discussion of the claims and rights pertinent to the case can be outlined.

1. Experimentation was performed on institutionalized, mentally retarded children;
2. The institution and maintenance of hepatitis serum banks (for the study of the natural history and prevention of the disease) used, as the most important source of specimens, the data from children whose infection was from the artificial exposure to the Willowbrook strains; and
3. The method of obtaining an "informed consent" was by the use of parental proxy consent.

The matter of informed consent is at the heart of the ethical problem raised by these experiments. What is informed consent and when does it properly apply? Lucille Kelly outlines the composition of an informed consent as follows:

1. explanation of the condition;
2. explanation of procedures to be used, including a discussion of the possible consequences;
3. discussion of alternate treatments;
4. discussion of the benefits to be expected though not assured;
5. an offer to answer patient's questions; and
6. an understanding that the patient is not being coerced to agree and that he may withdraw if he changes his mind.[3]

These stipulations are especially applicable to the therapeutic situation prior to surgery but they are not limited to that situation only.

Informed consent is also paramount in a second situation. It must be applied to the research methods used in today's experimentation, for example, blind and double blind studies, human therapeutic and nontherapeutic research. The Department of Health, Education, and Welfare's Policy on Protection of Human Subjects defines informed consent in these situations as "the agreement obtained from a subject, or from his authorized representative, to the subject's participation in an activity." The basic elements include:

1. a fair explanation of procedures to be followed, including an identification of those which are experimental;
2. a description of attendant risks, discomforts;
3. a description of the benefits to be expected;
4. a disclosure of appropriate alternative procedures that would be advantageous for the subject;
5. an offer to answer any questions concerning procedures; and,
6. instruction to subject to inform him that he is free to withdraw his consent and discontinue participation at any time.[4]

These are important elements to keep in mind as we consider the nontherapeutic research on the Willowbrook children.[5]

The issue of informed consent clearly involved the matter of patients' moral rights. Such rights are those one is thought to have a justifiable moral claim to enjoy. They always imply correlative duties on the part of another person or agent.[6] It is clear enough that researchers have to find ways to carry out important investigations for the common good, but it is also clear that they must be extremely careful not to abuse the moral rights of the subjects used in experimentation. Keeping in mind the question as to whether this case is one more directly relating to the rights of parents or the rights of children, let us consider a number of the basic moral rights involved in this case.

Right of Bodily Integrity

In medical care and research, the individual has the right and authority to accept or decline the treatment proposed when an intrusion on her or his person is necessary. We acknowledge this right by the use of informed consent.[7] In the Willowbrook studies, the children involved were subjected to intramuscular injections of infected serum or received the exposure via undiluted serum by mouth. In some instances following exposure evidence of liver dysfunction occurred.[8] It thus appears that the right of the Willowbrook patient was violated. Protection of this right is the crux of informed consent. Violation can be expressed as assault, battery, negligence, malpractice, and even trespassing.[9]

Right of Self-Determination

The protection of this second right is also an important consideration in the use of informed consent in therapeutic and nontherapeutic research. The subject must have full knowledge of what he or she is consenting to, must be entering the study voluntarily, and must be advised that he or she may withdraw at any time in the investigation.[10,11] There are examples of violation of the children's right of self-determination in the Willowbrook studies. Paul Ramsey describes an instance of questionable coercion of parents who wished to admit their children to the school.[12] In 1964, when the school was closed to admission because of overcrowding, new patients were continually accepted in the separate part of the institution which was carrying out the research. Applicants were placed on a waiting list but parents were informed that there were vacancies in the research unit if they wanted to volunteer their child for that. Can it be deduced from this account that the parents who admitted their children under this stipulation were doing so "voluntarily?"

The researchers give an extensive account of their consent method. They utilized many staff people (psychiatric social workers, private doctors, nurses, attendants) in a group technique of obtaining consent. Various meetings, briefing sessions, and tours were attended by those interested, and the "purposes, potential benefits, and potential hazards of the program" were discussed with parents.[13] But as Beecher points out, "nothing is said regarding what was told them concerning the appreciable hazards involved."[14] Did they have full knowledge of what they consented to?

In reference to the advisement of voluntary withdrawal at any time in the investigation, the researchers did state they informed parents that the consent could be withdrawn any time before the beginning of the particular program. But, could the children be withdrawn after artificial exposure was performed and then given proper care?

Rights of Minors and Incompetent Persons

The American Nurses' Association Guidelines on Ethical Values note that investigators must give particular attention to safeguarding these important rights in the case of the use of minors or incompetent persons in research.[15] In our case study, the subjects were institutionalized, mentally retarded children. Ramsey defends his thoughts on the wrongness of using children in homes for the retarded in nontherapeutic research because "they are a captive population."[16] He states that use of these children for "purely experimental purposes ought to be made legally impossible" by legally invalidating proxy consent for a child to procedures having no relation to his or her treatment.[17] From the depiction of this research study, could one say that it was designed to protect the mentally retarded children at Willowbrook?

From the above discussion, one can see that the rights of these subjects were not always rigorously protected throughout the investigation. This introduces the perception of the ethical problem: Did the legal guardians (parents) of these children receive a fully informed explanation of the research and did they freely give consent? Is it right to perform an experiment on normal or mentally retarded children when no benefit can result for them?

Clinical Data Pertinent to the Case

Krugman and Giles presented many justifications for doing the experiments. These included: (1) the hepatitis strain at Willowbrook was especially mild in three to ten year olds; (2) patients were naturally exposed to hepatitis and most new admissions become infected in the first six to twelve months; (3) subjects were admitted to a special isolation facility; (4) artificial induction of the virus implied a "therapeutic" effect because of the immunity conferred; (5) only children whose parents consented were included in the study;[18] wards of the state were not used, although the administrator at the school could have legally consented for them;[19] and (6) the studies were reviewed and sanctioned by such agencies as the committee on human experimentation of New York University (where Dr. Drugman held a faculty position) and the Armed Forces Epidemiological Board (which supported the contract).[20]

Do these facts justify performing the hepatitis research on the children? Was the exposure genuinely therapeutic? Were there obvious potential benefits accrued by the subjects? Was the parental consent adequate? It may be impossible to reach a completely satisfactory and universally accepted answer to these questions, but it is helpful to examine the relevant factors apparent in this case.

The first factor to consider is the use of nontherapeutic research. Fried defines this as experimentation carried out on a person solely to obtain information of use to others. It does not treat some illness which the subject may have.[21] It appears that the research done at Willowbrook does not qualify as therapeutic research by these standards. The testing of the neutralization of the infectivity of infectious hepatitis by gamma globulin was done, but only the control group received the vaccine prior to being artificially exposed. The children did not have the disease until the serum was given orally or parenterally to them. The children were used to test the vaccine's effectiveness in modifying the disease. The final observations were that gamma globulin was of limited value in preventing serum hepatitis while it will neutralize infectious hepatitis. The researchers stated these observations were "anticipated." If this was so, why were the children used as a means to an end in the nontherapeutic research?

The second relevant factor in this case is the use of children as the subjects. The use of children as research subjects presents ethical problems of public concern. Some experimentation requires the use of children for it to be valid in applying the findings to this population. An adult subject, in some cases, could not be used. It is necessary to continue research on pediatric patients to maintain and improve their quality of life. This can be done only by means of therapeutic research. The child's rights must be honored and she or he, her- or himself, must benefit from the research (for example, treatment done will, it is hoped, improve or cure her or him). Paul Ramsey states, "It is immoral to use children who can't themselves consent and who ought not to be presumed to consent to research unrelated to their treatment."[22]

The use of the mentally retarded as research subjects is the third factor to be considered. Does the use of the mentally retarded as subjects instead of normal children imply they were considered as subhuman? What is their status? Are not they entitled to the same rights as competent individuals? Even today, some states have provisions which largely consider or assume the retarded person to be without rights, and may deny him or her due process or equal protection of the law.[23]

A controlled group, such as the institutionalized, are tempting as subjects for research. The children in this study are residents in a state school. This is the fourth relevant factor. The use of the institutionalized, by the very nature of that condition, means that voluntary, informed consent may not be able to be obtained.

The final relevant factor is that of the doctrine of informed consent of the human subject in experimentation. It is often difficult to obtain a truly informed consent. For example, if the subject knows what the researcher is looking for or testing, the validity may be destroyed. Sometimes the subject cannot understand all of the details, hazards, and complexities of the research even though they are adequately explained. The children in the Willowbrook studies were not able to understand, but the appointed authorities who consented for the subjects, the parents, were presumed to have understood in order to have given a valid consent. Without this full understanding of the information, the consent has little meaning.

There are moral and ethical dilemmas that may arise in the area of informed consent when the subject is a minor. Was the parental consent in the study adequate? Can a parent legally consent to the child's participation in nontherapeutic research? Is it ethical to do so and under what conditions should they consent? Unfortunately, there is little guidance in present laws, regulations, and codes of ethics to assist one in answering these questions.

The child's authorized representatives are her or his parents or legal guardians, because she or he is a minor and may lack sufficient comprehension to give consent. Proxy consent is valid, but this extends only to those procedures which are necessary for the child's care (including treatment for illness or prophylactic measures). Legal parental consent for experimental therapeutic measures has been generally well-accepted as sufficient even without legal authority.[24] And, as Ramsey states, "To consent in place of a child means to consent in his behalf medically, i.e., for medical reasons and possible benefit to him."[25]

The use of children in nontherapeutic research presents a twofold dilemma: first, there is no legal basis for parental consent to such an undertaking, and, second, even if legal authority were clear, proper execution of that authority requires further definition and review to ensure that the best interests of the child are kept in mind.[26]

In the Willowbrook studies many factors may have impinged on the parental consent in the best interests of the child. Parents may have wanted institutionalization for other reasons than provision of adequate care for the child, e.g., economic stress, physical or mental frustration, the stigma of retardation, and consideration for the other children in the family.[27] They may have thought that the action of letting their children become research subjects did actually produce a "benefit" for them (special unit, the "therapeutic" effect of the artificial exposure). Were they told all of the features that might have affected their willingness to allow participation? Did the parents who applied for admission when the overcrowding occurred realize that placing the child in the school became contingent upon consenting to the child's participation in the research?

Two ethicists who have voiced differing opinions on the validity of proxy consent in nontherapeutic research on children are Ramsey and McCormick. Ramsey says parents cannot consent to this, regardless of the experiment's significance. To do so would "treat a child not as a child. . . ."[28] He says that McCormick treats the child as an adult when sanctioning proxy consent. McCormick states that the individual "ought also to take into account, realize, and make efforts in behalf of the lives of others also, for we are social beings. . . ."[29]

Ethical Issues Involved

From much of the content of the previous discussion, one can deduce the ethical issues involved in this case. The prominent issues include the use of mentally retarded children in research, the violation of the rights of these individuals, the legality and ethics of proxy consent in nontherapeutic experimentation, and the stipulations of a truly informed consent (voluntary and adequate knowledge of risks). Veatch outlines more issues pertaining to the consent in experimental situations which can be involved in this case also. These include: the relationship of therapeutic to nontherapeutic research, relation of subject risk to societal benefit, the right of the patient to be an experimental subject, and the researcher's responsibility for harmful consequences.[30]

Applicable Ethical Principles and Alternative Strategies
for Solution

In the discussion of this bioethical issue certain principles can apply. We may identify the principles of beneficence, justice, non-maleficence, and autonomy as germane in this analysis.

The principle of beneficence is one of the components of Frankena's theory of obligation. He lists four "oughts" to this principle: not to inflict harm or evil (highest in importance), to prevent harm, to remove evil, and to do or promote good.[31] According to the positive focus of this principle we are asked to do beneficial acts in order to assist others in improving their situation. It is our moral duty to promote good. Kant states that beneficence is a principle which we have a moral obligation to observe but leaves it up to the individual to choose when to apply it.[32] In the Willowbrook studies it has been demonstrated that the promotion of good was not the first considered action in the research design.

The equal and comparative treatment of individuals is the foundation in the principle of justice. This includes the equal distribution of both harms and benefits throughout all of society. The overuse of such populations as the poor or institutionalized (e.g., Willowbrook School students) is criticized as "an inequitable distribution of research risks."[33] Justice as fairness to the least advantaged becomes the categorical imperative in the Kantian tradition.

A third applicable principle is that of non-maleficence. This principle asks us to do no harm (of great relevance to health care professionals). This means that the health worker must not compound a patient's condition by causing more injury—"primum non nocere"—"first of all, do no harm." Veatch says this principle gives weight to avoiding harm over and above that given to the good which is produced.[34] Kant contends that we have a moral obligation to this principle of non-maleficence. In this case study, it can be applied to the protection of the human subjects involved, the children. Was this principle rigorously applied?

The final principle, autonomy, applies to this case study because the issue of informed consent is involved. For an act to be autonomous, it must be voluntary and without coercion, two elements of an informed consent. As was pointed out previously, the freedom of choice of what can or will happen to one's bodily integrity is problematic in institutions. At Willowbrook, did the parents, as legal representatives, have an autonomous avenue of choice when it came to consenting to the child's experimental participation? What about the child's own right of autonomy? What would he or she really have wanted? Is the magnitude of harm given to the small number of children balanced with the benefits of the studies for many other of the children, the staff, and society. We are morally obligated to minimize this risk of harm even if we may lose the end we are seeking. The researchers had a duty to protect the children's autonomy, but was this done?

Paul Ramsey gives a few solutions and alternatives to the endemic hepatitis at Willowbrook and to the use of children as research subjects.[35] He asks why the researchers did not try to control or defeat the endemic situation by more routine procedures, such as placing new admissions in facilities away from the infection while eradicating the infection in each building? It was implied that the new admissions likely were not carrying the infection. Why not, he asks, find the source? As to the research subjects, why were not any of the staff of nearly one thousand persons used when it was written that everyone was "naturally" exposed to the virus? These are among the realistic alternatives that could have been used to improve the conditions at Willowbrook, but instead, the investigators used clearly debatable methods to their own advantage. This raises another question: What kind of review did the committees of the armed forces and New York University actually provide.

It seems clear that there are grounds for concluding that the research done on the retarded children at Willowbrook was morally questionable. It is worthwhile to consider the problem in the light of philosophical ethics, especially the teaching of the utilitarian and the formalist (deontologic) schools.

The utilitarian view holds that the right act has the greatest utility. This position advocates maximizing the greatest good and least amount of harm for the greatest number of people. Each individual counts as one. In the issue of informed consent, utilitarianism weighs the risks to the human subject against benefits to the subject and to society.[36] Looking at the hepatitis studies, it can be deduced that the research done to gain new knowledge was justified from the ethics of utilitarianism: good consequences for the greater number of people. Robert Veatch notes that in experimentation, doing harm to a small number of children, but on a balance producing greater benefit for society, is morally defensible according to classical utilitarianism.[37] This view allows using patients in research.

In contrast, the formalist approach contends that the rightness or wrongness of an act depends on the nature of the act and whether it is in agreement with moral law or principle. The rightness of an act does not depend on its consequences. The formalist holds that the moral values of the individual are of major significance and requires that they must be consistently universal. The same judgment would be made regardless of time, place, or person involved in a given situation. This position differs from the utilitarian view which hold that there are standards for choosing, judging, and reasoning morally to help us decide whether an act is right.[38]

Immanuel Kant, the most famous ethicist in ethical formalism, provides us with guidance in testing the application of moral rules or principles by means of his unconditional commands or categorical imperatives. The moral principle at stake in informed consent in the discussed case study was addressed by Kant when he said that all members of humankind ought to treat each other as an end, and never as a means to an end.[39] In application of this rule to the research at Willowbrook, one can see that, indeed, the children were not valued in themselves, as persons, but for what statistical findings the researchers could get out of them in an attempt to validate their hypotheses. It is morally right to treat each child as a unique individual even if this does not promote the greatest balance of good (consequences) for the other students, staff, and humanity. Thus, the children should not have been used in the experimentation even though it provided an improvement in the vaccine for future patients and staff.

Ramsey states that if one overrides the view of the future good to be achieved in informed consent, it would make us "continually willing to use a subject in medical investigations as a mere means."[40] Ramsey holds that the determination of the rightness of an act is an important consideration, in addition to determining the benefits obtained in medical care or investigation. The outcome of the research (consequences) do not make the act morally correct. Beecher accurately states this in his article by saying: "An experiment is ethical or not at its inception; it does not become ethical 'post hoc'—ends do not justify means. There is no ethical distinction between ends and means."[41]

It has already been noted here that it was morally wrong to use these children in the experiments at Willowbrook in order to gain new knowledge about the disease and to improve the vaccine, gamma globulin. The researchers' findings, as published in the *Journal of the American Medical Association,* have probably benefited many other individuals, including myself, who have received gamma globulin for prophylactic reasons. If these investigations are not allowed because of the previously mentioned justifications, how will medical care continue to improve?

We may conclude with a number of suggestions for continuing benefits to humankind.

> We should provide for more stringent rulings on informed consent by the newly forming human rights and experimentation committees in order to use the subject as an end only, never a means, in research.
>
> There should be more exposure to medical ethics in physicians' training, since they are the main body of researchers in the health care system.
>
> Nurses should be acquainted with more information on bioethics in their training so that they also will consistently acknowledge the patient's rights and become more effective in the role of patient advocate.
>
> Therapeutic research should be used only as the means to gain new knowledge so that the patient will benefit from the treatment.

These are only a few ways in which we can continue research to improve medical care, but all are concerned for the rights of the individuals and are not using the subject as a means to an end.

Endnotes

1. Robert M. Veatch, *Case Studies in Medical Ethics* (Cambridge, Mass.: Harvard University Press, 1977), p. 275.
2. Saul Krugman and Joan P. Giles, "Viral Hepatitis: New Light on an Old Disease," *Journal of the American Medical Association* 212 (May 1970), pp. 1019–1021.
3. Lucille Young Kelly, "The Patient's Right to Know," *Nursing Outlook* 24 (January 1976), p. 28.
4. U. S., Department of Health, Education, and Welfare, *The Institutional Guide to DHEW Policy of Protection of Human Subjects,* Pubn. no. (NIH) 72–102 (December 1, 1971), p. 7.
5. Charles Lowe, Duane Alexander, and Barbara Miskin, "Nontherapeutic Research on Children: An Ethical Dilemma," *Journal of Pediatrics* 84 (April 1974), p. 468.
6. Veatch, *Medical Ethics.*
7. William T. Carpenter and Carol Langsner, "The Nurse's Role in Informed Consent," *Nursing Times* (3 July 1975), p. 1049.
8. Krugman and Giles, "Viral Hepatitis," pp. 1025–1026.
9. Norman Cantor, "A Patient's Decision to Decline Lifesaving Medical Treatment: Bodily Integrity vs. the Preservation of Life" in *Ethics in Medicine,* ed. S. Reiser, A. Dyck, and W. Curran (Cambridge, Mass.: MIT Press, 1977), p. 159.
10. Jeanne S. Berthold, "Advancement of Science and Technology while Maintaining Human Rights and Values," *Nursing Research* 18 (November-December 1969), p. 517.
11. "The Nurse in Research—ANA Guidelines on Ethical Values," *Nursing Research* 17 (March-April 1968), p. 106.
12. Paul Ramsey, *The Patient as Person* (New Haven: Yale University Press, 1970), p. 54, citing the *Medical Tribune,* February 20, 1967, p.23.
13. Krugman and Giles, "Viral Hepatitis," p. 1020.
14. Henry K. Beecher, "Ethics and Clinical Research," in *Ethics in Medicine,* ed. Reiser, Dyck, and Curran.
15. "The Nurse in Research—ANA Guidelines," p. 107.
16. Ramsey, *Patient as Person,* p. 41.
17. *Ibid.,* p. 54.
18. Krugman and Giles, "Viral Hepatitis," p. 1020.
19. Ramsey, *Patient as Person,* p. 53.
20. Veatch, *Medical Ethics,* p. 275.
21. Charles Fried, "Informed Consent and Medical Experimentation" in *Contemporary Issues in Bioethics,* ed. Tom L. Beauchamp and Leroy Walters (Encino, Calif.: Dickenson Publishing, 1978), p. 436.
22. Paul Ramsey, "Enforcement of Morals: Non-therapeutic Research on Children—A Reply to Richard McCormick," *Hastings Center Report* 6 (August 1976), p. 21.
23. Anne J. Davis and Mila A. Aroskar, *Ethical Dilemmas and Nursing Practice* (New York: Appleton-Century-Crofts, 1978), citing *The Decisive Decade,* The President's Committee on Mental Retardation, 1970.

24. Lowe, Alexander, and Miskin, "Nontherapeutic Research on Children," p. 468.
25. Ramsey, *Patient as Person*, p. 26.
26. Lowe, Alexander, and Miskin, "Nontherapeutic Research on Children," pp. 468, 470.
27. Davis and Aroskar, *Ethical Dilemmas*, p. 166.
28. Ramsey, "Enforcement of Morals," p. 21.
29. Richard McCormick, "Proxy Consent in the Experimental Situation" in *Contemporary Issues in Bioethics*.
30. Veatch, *Medical Ethics*, p. 267.
31. Davis and Aroskar, *Ethical Dilemmas*, p. 21, citing W. K. Frankena, *Ethics*, 2nd edition, p. 47.
32. *Ibid.*, p. 24.
33. Walters, "Bioethics as a Field of Ethics" in *Contemporary Issues in Bioethics*.
34. Veatch, *Medical Ethics*, p. 8.
35. Ramsey, *Patient as Person*, pp. 48–49.
36. Davis and Aroskar, *Ethical Dilemmas*, p. 73.
37. Veatch, *Medical Ethics*, p. 7.
38. Davis and Aroskar, *Ethical Dilemmas*, p. 22.
39. *Ibid.*, p. 80.
40. Ramsey, *Patient as Person*, p. 11.
41. Beecher, "Clinical Research," p. 293.

Appendices

Code for Nurses

American Nurses' Association

1. The nurse provides services with respect for human dignity and the uniqueness of the client unrestricted by considerations of social or economic status, personal attributes, or the nature of health problems.
2. The nurse safeguards the client's right to privacy by judiciously protecting information of a confidential nature.
3. The nurse acts to safeguard the client and the public when health care and safety are affected by the incompetent, unethical, or illegal practice of any person.
4. The nurse assumes responsibility and accountability for individual nursing judgments and actions.
5. The nurse maintains competence in nursing.
6. The nurse exercises informed judgment and uses individual competence and qualifications as criteria in seeking consultation, accepting responsibilities, and delegating nursing activities to others.
7. The nurse participates in activities that contribute to the ongoing development of the profession's body of knowledge.
8. The nurse participates in the profession's efforts to implement and improve standards of nursing.
9. The nurse participates in the profession's efforts to establish and maintain conditions of employment conducive to high quality nursing care.

10. The nurse participates in the profession's effort to protect the public from misinformation and misrepresentation and to maintain the integrity of nursing.

11. The nurse collaborates with members of the health professions and other citizens in promoting community and national efforts to meet the health needs of the public.

Human Rights Guidelines for Nurses in Clinical and Other Research

American Nurses' Association

Ethical Guidelines

Nursing Activities and Ethical Issues

The need for protection of human rights potentially involves all activities that go beyond the established and accepted practices of the professional group involved. In health care practice, the need for protection of human rights is of singular importance for any and all activities when the focus is not specifically directed toward meeting the needs of the individual patient or subject. The development and refinement of scientific knowledge in nursing will increasingly involve nurses in clinical investigations with an emphasis on furthering knowledge rather than specifically on meeting patients' needs. Other nurses in their roles as practitioners in hospitals and other institutional settings can find themselves engaged in clinical research developed and implemented by practitioners in other fields. In both cases, ethical concerns about the potential violations of human rights become crucial whenever new and untried techniques and procedures are to be used and when the probable outcomes are unknown or doubtful.

Whenever nurses perform activities that are components of clinical research (whether directed by physicians, nurses, or other investigators), the need for protection of human rights must extend to the practitioners who are expected to participate in new and untried practices as well as to the subjects who are recipients of them. The concept of informed consent applies not only to subjects *per se* but also to any workers who are expected as part of their daily work to implement activities that potentially or actually carry risk for others or have uncertain outcomes.

Implementation of this guideline implies the need for written statements about conditions of employment and any special expectations about work performance above and beyond that usually expected of a person occupying the position of nurse. In advance of such employment, nurses need to know if they will be expected to provide medicines, treatments, and other procedures as part of double blind investigations. They need to know in advance if the work requires them to function as data-collectors for research in addition to their roles as nurses engaged in the delivery of patient care services. Conditions of employment must also provide for the option of not participating in clinical research if these work expectations are not spelled out in advance of employment.

Stated in a more general way, conditions of employment in settings in which clinical and/or other research is in progress need to be spelled out in detail for all potential workers. As a corollary, it follows that anyone employed in work that carries the potential of risk to others needs to be advised as to the types of risks involved, the ways of recognizing when risk is present, and the proper actions to take to counteract harmful effects and unnecessary danger.

Human Rights

Right to Freedom from Intrinsic Risk of Injury. In situations in which the nature of the activities or research design exposes an individual to increased possibility of emotional, social, or physical injury, the degree of risk needs to be estimated and specified by the principal investigator or his designate. It is incumbent upon all practitioners to recognize that risk is potentially present in all situations when novel and untried procedures are involved and there is little if any data upon which to predict outcomes. The primary problem faced by the investigator or practitioner is prediction of the extent of risk to the individual in comparison to the potential clinical benefit to him and/or the humanitarian importance of the knowledge to be gained.

In all instances, the prospective subject must be given all relevant information prior to participation in activities that go beyond established and accepted procedures necessary to meet his personal needs. By virtue of their calling, practitioners in the health professions seek to protect individuals under their care from arbitrary physical or mental suffering. Nurses must be increasingly vigilant in their concern for subjects and patients who by reason of their situation and/or illness are not able to protect themselves effectively from externally imposed threat or injury. They must also be sensitive to the tendency toward exploitation of "captive" populations such as students, patients in institutions, and prisoners.

Right of Privacy and Dignity. Human beings vary in their values and judgments about what is considered invasion of privacy and a threat to dignity through demeaning or dehumanizing conditions. The investigator cannot presume to decide for the other person on this matter of privacy and dignity. Consequently all proposals, investigative instruments, protocols, and techniques to be used in the particular activities need to be specified and discussed with the prospective subject and with any workers who are expected to participate in the activity as subjects, as data-collectors, or as both.

Consideration must be given to the development of safeguards such that no unanticipated physical, psychological, or social disadvantage accrues to subjects either during the study or as a result of dissemination of the findings. If the subject agrees voluntarily to share certain specific information about himself which he may or may not choose to divulge to others in a different context, then the investigator must provide assurance that the subject's anonymity will be protected. Specific prior consent must be obtained whenever the plan of a study or a report of findings sacrifices subject anonymity or confidentiality.

Special mechanisms for safeguarding the confidentiality of information must be developed whenever the information will not always remain under the control of the investigator. Potentially demeaning or dehumanizing conditions merit special consideration from both practitioners and investigators inasmuch as they are in many instances difficult to specify and to protect against. Health care practitioners need to be aware that violations involving human dignity have many potential long range repercussions when significant values of the individual are involved.

Subjects

The persons for whom human rights guidelines apply include all individuals involved in the activities described before. When activities are supported either directly or indirectly by government and other funding resources, the persons to whom these guidelines apply include the following groups: patients; out-patients; donors of organs, tissues, and services; informants; normal volunteers including students; and volunteers in groups with limited civil freedom. The latter classification refers to prisoners, residents or clients in institutions for the mentally ill and mentally retarded, and persons subject to military discipline, all of whom tend easily to fall into the class of captive audience and population vulnerable to exploitation.

The choice of minors and groups with limited civil freedom as research subjects can be justified, in most instances, only if there are benefits that will accrue in the future to them or to others in similar situations or classes. Strict standards governing the use of minors and other groups (including the unborn and the dead) lacking the capacity to give informed consent are being established with increasing frequency by various government statutes and regulations.

Society's Obligation and the Public Good

In a democratic society the rights of the individual are of necessity counter-balanced by actions and activities designed for the common good of collective man. Established public health practices such as the immunization of children against diphtheria and pertussis and the chlorination of public water supplies to prevent epidemics of water-borne disease are examples of societal actions in which personal rights gave way to collective rights for the benefit of society as a whole. These and many other public health practices came into being as a result of research seeking ways to treat and control disease.

Advancement of knowledge about health and health-promoting practices is also of value to society as a whole. So too is knowledge about patient responses and adaptations to illness and the effects of different nursing interventions on these responses and adaptations. Just as nurses have an obligation to protect the human rights of patients, so do they also have an obligation to support the accrual of knowledge that broadens the scientific underpinnings of nursing practice and the delivery of nursing services. Professional responsibility includes a recognition that research by qualified nurses is a resource in need of support and encouragement.

Mechanisms for Protection of Rights

Assurance—Informed Consent

On some occasions, a research design involves procedures or possible outcomes that may impinge upon the rights of someone related to the subject, such as a spouse or parent. In such cases the informed consent of that individual must also be obtained.

The informed consent of parents or legal guardians must be obtained for investigations that involve minors or individuals judged to be legally incompetent to handle their own affairs. In instances in which these subjects have the capacity to comprehend the implications of the proposed activity, they should also be asked to give their consent. In this case, consent supplements rather than supplants that of the parent or other legal agent.

As part of any study protocol, documentation of the procedures to be followed in obtaining informed consent is expected. If written consent is not to be obtained, justification of the omission must be provided. Since the investigator carries the major responsibility for insuring that the rights of the subject are protected, he must throughout the course of the investigation and thereafter scrupulously adhere to the mutual agreement (whether oral or written) contracted with each subject.

Assurance—Institutions and Agencies

There is increasing public support for systematic accountability to insure that unintentional professional and/or investigator bias does not overtly or covertly deny individuals their rights. In almost all circumstances, either the professional nurse or the prospective subject is under the aegis of an institution or agency, and the institution is responsible for establishing and maintaining procedures to safeguard human rights. In most instances, the protective mechanism takes place through a committee judged competent to review projects and other activities that involve human subjects. Membership on the review committee should be representative of all occupational groups (including practicing nurses) whose members are likely to be involved either directly or indirectly in the implementation of the activities or projects undertaken.

In most institutions, the committee is responsible for an initial and continuing review and approval of each activity deemed necessary for review. The review is designed to determine and assure that subject rights have been protected, that the procedures proposed for obtaining informed consent are adequate, that appropriate records are maintained regarding the selection, participation, and protection of subjects, and that circumstances that may or do adversely affect the rights or the welfare of individual subjects are reviewed and acted upon appropriately. In addition, when projects are supported by government funds, the institution must also provide for appropriate professional attention in case the subject suffers physical, psychological, or other injury as a result of participation in the particular activity. In some institutions investigators must also explain how and when identifying data are to be destroyed when the study has been completed.

There are investigational areas in which, by the nature of the data used and the manipulations applied to it, consent by subjects is not required. This ruling would apply to stored data, information, tissue, body fluids, or other materials obtained in the course of routine, professional or clinical observations and activities, and collection does not involve any increased risk to the subject. According to societal values as represented by the federal government, however, use of any of these items for many research, training, and service purposes may present psychological, sociological, or legal risks to the subject or his authorized representative. Determination of whether such risks are involved and whether the use of the materials is within the scope of the original consent is a responsibility of the institution through its established review committee.

In clinical studies that involve hospital or other institutional staff in addition to the research team, special precautions are needed to safeguard the human rights of these employees. If the research design requires actions by persons who are not regular members of the research staff (such as nurses assigned to a clinical unit), steps must be taken to insure that these persons are informed about the procedures and activities expected of them. Responsibility for obtaining informed consent to participate in research belongs to the principal investigator and must not be delegated to regular employees of the institution for the sake of convenience. So that all members of the institutional staff can know that research is in progress, a copy of the patient's (consumer's) signed consent form should be attached as part of that patient's (consumer's) hospital record.

To monitor the utilization of both patients and nursing personnel in research and other special activities, a list of all research projects approved by the institutional review committee must be sent routinely to nursing and other departments that are likely to be involved in the implementation of the studies. Conversely, to safeguard the overutilization of patients and nursing personnel in research and other special projects and to provide a mechanism for approving research and special activities within departments of nursing, organized nursing services have responsibility to develop and enforce written policies and guidelines governing these matters with special attention to protection of the rights of prospective subjects. Guidelines designed to protect human subjects against violation of their rights must incorporate explicit directions for protecting the highly vulnerable individuals who for one or more reasons have difficulty in providing informed consent. High risk individuals include but may not be limited to those who are illiterate, lack command of the English language (or other primary language), do not recognize their right to refuse participation without jeopardizing their care, or for some reason are unable to comprehend instructions or directions.

The institution also has responsibility to formulate mechanisms and procedures for the reporting of events in which human rights are violated. Such mechanisms and procedures need to be brought to the attention of all members of the staff and all consumers of services. The mechanism of reporting should be such that the rights of the person reporting the event also are not violated.

Assurance—Professions

Increased use of hospitals and health care facilities for clinical and other research means that practicing nurses in many institutions are knowingly or unknowingly serving as participants in research designed and implemented by others. Increased educational opportunity for nurses has produced a corps of nurse researchers who are actively engaged in scientific study. Yet stereotyped images of nurses and nursing have in some settings obstructed active participation by nurses on institutional committees for review of research. The profession of nursing through its organization, the American Nurses' Association, has an obligation to publicly support the inclusion of nurses as regular members of institutional review committees and to make this policy known through written statements of policy.

Because nurses in practice encounter many patients whose rights can unknowingly or inadvertently be violated, the profession of nursing through its national organization carries additional responsibility for the development of written policies and guidelines governing the rights of human subjects to guide nurses at many different levels of practice in formulating policies and procedures pertaining to these matters in their own jurisdictions. The professional nurse's responsibility for protecting the rights of human subjects requires that mechanisms be established whereby violations of rights can be reported and actions taken to countermand the violations. The profession of nursing through its organization at the state level has responsibility to develop mechanisms whereby grievances of nurses may be reported and redressed when these nurses have knowledge of violation of human rights.

Personal Responsibility

In order for nursing to fulfill its professional obligations in a rapidly changing society, each nurse must develop an awareness of the issues and a framework for dealing effectively with emerging human rights problems. Ethical issues frequently involve conflicting values, and in many individual cases ethical standards are not specified in sufficient clarity to allow for unambiguous decision-making. As knowledgeable participants in health care practice and research, professional nurses should involve themselves in institutional policy making and review committee activities.

As knowledgeable participants, nurses need also to become informed about various legal parameters affecting practitioner-client relationships. With respect to human rights, legal accountability focuses upon evidence that the professional practitioner or researcher has not failed his/her responsibility by either intentionally or unintentionally withholding relevant information that might have altered the patient or subject's decision. Knowledge about the changing scope of nursing responsibility and the emerging ethical issues affecting all practitioners in health care today is a necessary requirement for professional nursing practice in which accountability for the protection of human rights of consumers is accepted.

A Patient's Bill of Rights

American Hospital Association

The American Hospital Association Board of Trustees' Committee on Health Care for the Disadvantaged, which has been a consistent advocate on behalf of consumers of health care services, developed the Statement on a Patient's Bill of Rights, which was approved by the AHA House of Delegates February 6, 1973. The statement was published in several forms, one of which was the S74 leaflet in the Association's S series. The S74 leaflet is now superseded by this reprinting of the statement.

The American Hospital Association presents a Patient's Bill of Rights with the expectation that observance of these rights will contribute to more effective patient care and greater satisfaction for the patient, his physician, and the hospital organization. Further, the Association presents these rights in the expectation that they will be supported by the hospital on behalf of its patients, as an integral part of the healing process. It is recognized that a personal relationship between the physician and the patient is essential for the provision of proper medical care. The traditional physician-patient relationship takes on a new dimension when care is rendered within an organizational structure. Legal precedent has established that the institution itself also has a responsibility to the patient. It is in recognition of these factors that these rights are affirmed.

1. The patient has the right to considerate and respectful care.

2. The patient has the right to obtain from his physician complete current information concerning his diagnosis, treatment, and prognosis in terms the patient can be reasonably expected to understand. When it is not medically advisable to give such information to the patient, the information should be made available to an appropriate person in his behalf. He has the right to know, by name, the physician responsible for coordinating his care.

3. The patient has the right to receive from his physician information necessary to give informed consent prior to the start of any procedure and/or treatment. Except in emergencies, such information for informed consent should include but not necessarily be limited to the specific procedure and/or treatment, the medically significant risks involved, and the probable duration of incapacitation. Where medically significant alternatives for care or treatment exist, or when the patient requests information concerning medical alternatives, the patient has the right to such information. The patient also has the right to know the name of the person responsible for the procedures and/or treatment.

4. The patient has the right to refuse treatment to the extent permitted by law and to be informed of the medical consequences of his action.

5. The patient has the right to every consideration of his privacy concerning his own medical care program. Case discussion, consultation, examination, and treatment are confidential and should be conducted discreetly. Those not directly involved in his care must have the permission of the patient to be present.

6. The patient has the right to expect that all communications and records pertaining to his care should be treated as confidential.

7. The patient has the right to expect that within its capacity a hospital must make reasonable response to the request of a patient for services. The hospital must provide evaluation, service, and/or referral as indicated by the urgency of the case. When medically permissible, a patient may be transferred to another facility only after he has received complete information and explanation concerning the needs for and alternatives to such a transfer. The institution to which the patient is to be transferred must first have accepted the patient for transfer.

8. The patient has the right to obtain information as to any relationship of his hospital to other health care and educational institutions insofar as his care is concerned. The patient has the right to obtain information as to the existence of any professional relationships among individuals, by name, who are treating him.

9. The patient has the right to be advised if the hospital proposes to engage in or perform human experimentation affecting his care or treatment. The patient has the right to refuse to participate in such research projects.

10. The patient has the right to expect reasonable continuity of care. He has the right to know in advance what appointment times and physicians are available

and where. The patient has the right to expect that the hospital will provide a mechanism whereby he is informed by his physician or a delegate of the physician of the patient's continuing health care requirements following discharge.

11. The patient has the right to examine and receive an explanation of his bill regardless of source of payment.

12. The patient has the right to know what hospital rules and regulations apply to his conduct as a patient.

No catalog of rights can guarantee for the patient the kind of treatment he has a right to expect. A hospital has many functions to perform, including the prevention and treatment of disease, the education of both health professionals and patients, and the conduct of clinical research. All these activities must be conducted with an overriding concern for the patient, and, above all, the recognition of his dignity as a human being. Success in achieving this recognition assures success in the defense of the rights of the patient.

Code for Nurses:
Ethical Concepts Applied to Nursing

International Council of Nurses

The fundamental responsibility of the nurse is fourfold: to promote
health, to prevent illness, to restore health and to alleviate suffering.
The need for nursing is universal. Inherent in nursing is respect for life,
dignity and rights of man. It is unrestricted by considerations of na-
tionality, race, creed, colour, age, sex, politics or social status.
Nurses render health services to the individual, the family and the community and coordinate their services with those of related groups.

Nurses and People

The nurse's primary responsibility is to those people who require nursing
care.
The nurse, in providing care, promotes an environment in which the
values, customs and spiritual beliefs of the individual are respected.
The nurse holds in confidence personal information and uses judgement in
sharing this information.

Nurses and Practice

The nurse carries personal responsibility for nursing practice and for
maintaining competence by continual learning.
The nurse maintains the highest standards of nursing care possible within
the reality of a specific situation.

The nurse uses judgement in relation to individual competence when accepting and delegating responsibilities.

The nurse when acting in a professional capacity should at all times maintain standards of personal conduct which reflect credit upon the profession.

Nurses and Society

The nurse shares with other citizens the responsibility for initiating and supporting action to meet the health and social needs of the public.

Nurses and Co-Workers

The nurse sustains a cooperative relationship with co-workers in nursing and other fields.

The nurse takes appropriate action to safeguard the individual when his care is endangered by a co-worker or any other person.

Nurses and the Profession

The nurse plays the major role in determining and implementing desirable standards of nursing practice and nursing education.

The nurse is active in developing a core of professional knowledge.

The nurse, acting through the professional organization, participates in establishing and maintaining equitable social and economic working conditions in nursing.

The Nuremberg Code

The great weight of the evidence before us is to the effect that certain types of medical experiments on human beings, when kept within reasonably well-defined bounds, conform to the ethics of the medical profession generally. The protagonists of the practice of human experimentation justify their views on the basis that such experiments yield results for the good of society that are unprocurable by other methods or means of study. All agree, however, that certain basic principles must be observed in order to satisfy moral, ethical and legal concepts.

1. The voluntary consent of the human subject is absolutely essential.

This means that the person involved should have legal capacity to give consent; should be so situated as to be able to exercise free power of choice, without the intervention of any element of force, fraud, deceit, duress, overreaching, or other ulterior form of constraint or coercion; and should have sufficient knowledge and comprehension of the elements of the subject matter involved as to enable him to make an understanding and enlightened decision. This latter element requires that before the acceptance of an affirmative decision by the experimental subject there should be made known to him the nature, duration, and purpose of the experiment; the method and means by which it is to be conducted; all inconveniences and hazards reasonably to be expected; and the

From *Trials of War Criminals Before the Nuremberg Military Tribunals Under Control Council Law No. 10,* Vol. II, Nuremberg, October 1946–April 1949.

effects upon his health or person which may possibly come from his participation in the experiment.

The duty and responsibility for ascertaining the quality of the consent rests upon each individual who initiates, directs or engages in the experiment. It is a personal duty and responsibility which may not be delegated to another with impunity.

2. The experiment should be such as to yield fruitful results for the good of society, unprocurable by other methods or means of study, and not random and unnecessary in nature.

3. The experiment should be so designed and based on the results of animal experimentation and a knowledge of the natural history of the disease or other problem under study that the anticipated results will justify the performance of the experiment.

4. The experiment should be so conducted as to avoid all unnecessary physical and mental suffering and injury.

5. No experiment should be conducted where there is an *a priori* reason to believe that death or disabling injury will occur; except, perhaps, in those experiments where the experimental physicians also serve as subjects.

6. The degree of risk to be taken should never exceed that determined by the humanitarian importance of the problem to be solved by the experiment.

7. Proper preparations should be made and adequate facilities provided to protect the experimental subject against even remote possibilities of injury, disability, or death.

8. The experiment should be conducted only by scientifically qualified persons. The highest degree of skill and care should be required through all stages of the experiment of those who conduct or engage in the experiment.

9. During the course of the experiment the human subject should be at liberty to bring the experiment to an end if he has reached the physical or mental state where continuation of the experiment seems to him to be impossible.

10. During the course of the experiment the scientist in charge must be prepared to terminate the experiment at any stage, if he has probable cause to believe, in the exercise of the good faith, superior skill and careful judgment required of him that a continuation of the experiment is likely to result in injury, disability, or death to the experimental subject.

Declaration of Helsinki

World Medical Association

Introduction

It is the mission of the medical doctor to safeguard the health of the people. His or her knowledge and conscience are dedicated to the fulfillment of this mission.

The Declaration of Geneva of The World Medical Association binds the doctor with the words "The health of my patient will be my first consideration," and the International Code of Medical Ethics declares that, "Any act or advice which could weaken physical or mental resistance of a human being may be used only in his interest."

The purpose of biomedical research involving human subjects must be to improve diagnostic, and therapeutic and prophylactic procedures and the understanding of the aetiology and pathogenesis of disease.

In current medical practice most diagnostic, therapeutic or prophylactic procedures involve hazards. This applies *a fortiori* to biomedical research.

Medical progress is based on research which ultimately must rest in part on experimentation involving human subjects.

In the field of biomedical research a fundamental distinction must be recognized between medical research in which the aim is essentially diagnostic or

Recommendations guiding medical doctors in biomedical research involving human subjects. Adopted by the 18th World Medical Assembly, Helsinki, Finland, 1964, and revised by the 29th World Medical Assembly, Tokyo, Japan, October 1975. Reprinted with permission of the World Medical Association, Inc. from the "Declaration of Helsinki," revised edition.

therapeutic for a patient, and medical research, the essential object of which is purely scientific and without direct diagnostic or therapeutic value to the person subjected to the research.

Special caution must be exercised in the conduct of research which may affect the environment, and the welfare of animals used for research must be respected.

Because it is essential that the results of laboratory experiments be applied to human beings to further scientific knowledge and to help suffering humanity, The World Medical Association has prepared the following recommendations as a guide to every doctor in biomedical research involving human subjects. They should be kept under review in the future. It must be stressed that the standards as drafted are only a guide to physicians all over the world. Doctors are not relieved from criminal, civil and ethical responsibilities under the laws of their own countries.

I. Basic Principles

1. Biomedical research involving human subjects must conform to generally accepted scientific principles and should be based on adequately performed laboratory and animal experimentation and on a thorough knowledge of the scientific literature.

2. The design and performance of each experimental procedure involving human subjects should be clearly formulated in an experimental protocol which should be transmitted to a specially appointed independent committee for consideration, comment and guidance.

3. Biomedical research involving human subjects should be conducted only by scientifically qualified persons and under the supervision of a clinically competent medical person. The responsibility for the human subject must always rest with a medically qualified person and never rest on the subject of research, even though the subject has given his or her consent.

4. Biomedical research involving human subjects cannot legitimately be carried out unless the importance of the objective is in proportion to the inherent risk to the subject.

5. Every biomedical research project involving human subjects should be preceded by careful assessment of predictable risks in comparison with foreseeable benefits to the subject or to others. Concern for the interests of the subject must always prevail over the interests of science and society.

6. The right of the research subject to safeguard his or her integrity must always be respected. Every precaution should be taken to respect the privacy of the subject and to minimize the impact of the study on the subject's physical and mental integrity and on the personality of the subject.

7. Doctors should abstain from engaging in research projects involving human subjects unless they are satisfied that the hazards involved are believed to be

predictable. Doctors should cease any investigation if the hazards are found to outweigh the potential benefits.

8. In publication of the results of his or her research, the doctor is obliged to preserve the accuracy of the results. Reports of experimentation not in accordance with the principles laid down in this Declaration should not be accepted for publication.

9. In any research on human beings, each potential subject must be adequately informed of the aims, methods, anticipated benefits and potential hazards of the study and the discomfort it may entail. He or she should be informed that he or she is at liberty to abstain from participation in the study and that he or she is free to withdraw his or her consent to participation at any time. The doctor should then obtain the subject's freely-given informed consent, preferably in writing.

10. When obtaining informed consent for the research project the doctor should be particularly cautious if the subject is in a dependent relationship to him or her or may consent under duress. In that case the informed consent should be obtained by a doctor who is not engaged in the investigation and who is completely independent of this official relationship.

11. In case of legal incompetence, informed consent should be obtained from the legal guardian in accordance with national legislation. Where physical or mental incapacity makes it impossible to obtain informed consent, or when the subject is a minor, permission from the responsible relative replaces that of the subject in accordance with national legislation.

12. The research protocol should always contain a statement of the ethical considerations involved and should indicate that the principles enunciated in the present Declaration are complied with.

II. Medical Research Combined with Professional Care
(Clinical Research)

1. In the treatment of the sick person, the doctor must be free to use a new diagnostic and therapeutic measure, if in his or her judgement it offers hope of saving life, reestablishing health or alleviating suffering.

2. The potential benefits, hazards and discomfort of a new method should be weighed against the advantages of the best current diagnostic and therapeutic methods.

3. In any medical study, every patient—including those of a control group, if any—should be assured of the best proven diagnostic and therapeutic method.

4. The refusal of the patient to participate in a study must never interfere with the doctor–patient relationship.

5. If the doctor considers it essential not to obtain informed consent, the specific reasons for this proposal should be stated 'n the expe-imental protocol for transmission to the independent committee (I, 2).

6. The doctor can combine medical research with professional care, the objective being the acquisition of new medical knowledge, only to the extent that medical research is justified by its potential diagnostic or therapeutic value for the patient.

III. Non-therapeutic Biomedical Research Involving Human Subjects (Non-Clinical Biomedical Research)

1. In the purely scientific application of medical research carried out on a human being, it is the duty of the doctor to remain the protector of the life and health of that person on whom biomedical research is being carried out.

2. The subjects should be volunteers—either healthy persons or patients for whom the experimental design is not related to the patient's illness.

3. The investigator or the investigating team should discontinue the research if in his/her or their judgement it may, if continued, be harmful to the individual.

4. In research on man, the interest of science and society should never take precedence over considerations related to the well-being of the subject.

Index